Wilson's Practical Meat Inspection

Sixth Edition

Andrew Wilson
MRCVS, DVSM
Examiner in Meat Inspection for
The Royal Society of Health

Revised by

William Wilson
MCIEH
Honorary Lecturer at
The University of Birmingham

b

Blackwell
Science

© 1968, 1975, 1980, 1985, 1991, 1998 by
Blackwell Science Ltd
Editorial Offices:
Osney Mead, Oxford OX2 0EL
25 John Street, London WC1N 2BL
23 Ainslie Place, Edinburgh EH3 6AJ
350 Main Street, Malden
   MA 02148 5018, USA
54 University Street, Carlton
   Victoria 3053, Australia

Other Editorial Offices:

Blackwell Wissenschafts-Verlag GmbH
Kurfürstendamm 57
10707 Berlin, Germany

Blackwell Science KK
MG Kodenmacho Building
7-10 Kodenmacho Nihombashi
Chuo-ku, Tokyo 104, Japan

First published 1968
Second edition 1975
Third edition 1980
Fourth edition 1985
Fifth edition 1991
Reprinted 1997
Sixth edition 1998

Set in 10/13pt Times
by DP Photosetting, Aylesbury, Bucks
Printed and bound in Great Britain by
MPG Books Limited, Bodmin, Cornwall

DISTRIBUTORS

Marston Book Services Ltd
PO Box 269
Abingdon
Oxon OX14 4YN
(*Orders:* Tel: 01235 465500
          Fax: 01235 465555)

USA
Blackwell Science, Inc.
Commerce Place
350 Main Street
Malden, MA 02148 5018
(*Orders:* Tel: 800 759 6102
          617 388 8250
          Fax: 617 388 8255)

Canada
Copp Clark Professional
200 Adelaide Street West, 3rd Floor
Toronto, Ontario M5H 1W7
(*Orders:* Tel: 416 597 1616
          800 815 9417
          Fax: 416 597 1617)

Australia
Blackwell Science Pty Ltd
54 University Street
Carlton, Victoria 3053
(*Orders:* Tel: 03 9347 0300
          Fax: 03 934 5001)

A catalogue record for this title is available
from the British Library

ISBN 0-632-04898-0

Library of Congress
Cataloging-in-Publication Data
Wilson, Andrew
   Practical meat inspection/Andrew Wilson.
   – 6th ed./revised by William Wilson.
      p.   cm.
   Includes index.
   ISBN 0-632-04898-0
   1. Meat inspection.   I. Wilson, William,
MCIEH.   II. Title.
TS1975.W56   1997
664′.907–dc21
                              97-20711
                                   CIP

Contents

Preface to Sixth Edition   v
Preface to First Edition   vi

1 Cells and tissues   1
2 Deer and venison   6

Systems of the Body   9

3 Skeletal system   11
4 Muscular system   23
5 Circulatory system   24
6 Lymphatic system   31
7 Respiratory system   42
8 Digestive system   48
9 Urogenital system   62
10 Nervous system   71
11 Endocrine system   75

Slaughter and Age/Sex Determination   79

12 The slaughter of animals   81
13 Sex characteristics and estimation of age   89

Pathology and Judgement in Disease   97

14 Abnormal and general pathological conditions   99
15 Specific diseases   115
16 Parasitic diseases   140
17 Affections of specific parts and tumours   167

Butchers' Joints and Meat Products   195

18 Butchers' joints   197
19 Meat preservation and meat products   202
20 Food poisoning from meat products   225

Rabbits   229

21 Diseases of rabbits   231

Poultry   **235**

22 Sex and age characteristics of poultry   237
23 Anatomy of the fowl   241
24 Slaughter and dressing of poultry   256
25 Diseases of poultry   261
26 Affections of specific parts of poultry   278

Appendix 1: Legislation   282
Appendix 2: Colloquial terms   283

Bibliography   286

Index   287

Colour plate section following page 122.

Preface to Sixth Edition

The contents have been updated to reflect legislative changes, improved knowledge of particular diseases such as BSE, *E. coli* O157, and developments in animal welfare and husbandry since the fifth edition. Additional photographic plates of diseases for both red and poultry meat have been included. The poultry section has been enlarged giving more detail concerning the sexing and ageing of poultry. I am grateful for the technical knowledge and assistance given by my colleague Mr R. Butler *MSc, BA Hons, BA, CIEH*. I would also like to add my thanks to my wife, Stephanie, for her encouragement, support and constructive input.

William Wilson

Dedication

I wish to dedicate this edition to my late father, Andrew Wilson. His knowledge and foresight in producing the first five editions of this book have provided a firm foundation for this revision, the sixth edition. God bless you, Dad.

Preface to First Edition

This book is based on a course of lectures on meat inspection, and is intended for all those interested in the practical aspects of the subject, particularly veterinary students, trainee public health inspectors and trainee meat inspectors. While the sections dealing with physiology and anatomy have been deliberately made somewhat elementary they do provide all the information required by meat inspectors, while veterinary students, and to a lesser degree, public health inspectors, learn these subjects as a separate part of their course.

I have tried to deal comprehensively with meat inspection, but it must be stressed that it is essentially a practical subject which cannot be learned from books alone. I have, however, designed both text and illustrations to emphasise all the important facts which students should remember, excluding all irrelevant material.

It is most important that students should familiarise themselves with normal tissues so that when something abnormal turns up it can be recognised.

In writing this book I have had much helpful criticism from colleagues in Birmingham; in particular from Mr George E. Bousfield *MAPHI*. I am most grateful for his help. I also wish to thank Mr Jack Baker *FRSH*, for the section on preservation by heat, and Mr Donald J. Knight, meat inspector, for the section on bacon curing and meat products.

Chapter 1
Cells and Tissues

Physiology is the study of the various activities of living organisms. Such activities include:

(1) Assimilation of food and oxygen to produce energy necessary for existence
(2) Excretion of waste products
(3) Growth
(4) Reproduction.

All living organisms are composed of cells, the form of which can be seen microscopically. The simplest form of life is composed of only one cell, e.g. the amoeba. Most animals, however, are made of a great number of cells and tissues. Each tissue has its own particular type of cell, e.g. muscle cells differ in size and shape from those of the liver. Basically each cell has the same structure (Fig. 1.1).

Cells

A cell consists of *protoplasm* enclosed within a *cell membrane*. The protoplasm contains a *nucleus* which is surrounded by *cytoplasm*. Mammalian red blood cells are unusual in that they do not contain nuclei.

The nucleus consists of a *nuclear membrane*, *nucleoplasm* and *nucleolus*. The nuclear membrane is a perforated structure which separates the nucleus from the cytoplasm. The nucleoplasm contains the chromosomes which are constructed mainly of deoxyribonucleic acid (DNA), and the nucleolus is rich in ribonucleic acid (RNA).

The cytoplasm contains many living inclusions:

(1) *Mitochondria*. These are found in most abundance in situations where there is great activity, e.g. in the muscles. They are concerned with the conversion of adenosine diphosphate (ADP) to the triphosphate form (ATP) for energy purposes.
(2) *Ribosomes*. These are the site of protein synthesis.
(3) *Golgi bodies*. These are involved in the production of enzymes and hormones.
(4) *Lysosomes*. These break down food particles.

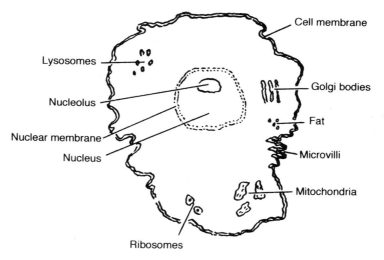

Fig. 1.1 Animal cell.

The cytoplasm also contains non-living inclusions, such as fat and glycogen.
Cells are constantly dying and being replaced by new cells, e.g. the red blood cell cycle is about 14 days.

Tissues

The animal body is composed of tissues. The main tissues are: epithelial, connective, muscular, blood, lymphatic and nervous.

Epithelial tissues

These cover the free surfaces of the body. There are various types:

(1) *Stratified epithelium* is many cells thick. It covers the anterior surface of the cornea and forms the epidermis of the skin, the superficial cells of which are dead, flattened and scale-like, whereas the deeper cells are polyhedral and columnar in shape.

(2) *Transitional epithelium* is a type of stratified epithelium that has only three or four layers of cells. Most of the urinary tract has this type of epithelium.

(3) *Pavement epithelium* covers the unexposed parts of the body, e.g. the pleural and peritoneal cavities, and the blood and lymph vessels.

(4) *Columnar epithelium* is a more active type of epithelium and is found lining the stomach and intestines.

(5) *Ciliated epithelium* is found in the lungs and trachea, in the fallopian tubes, uterus and efferent tubes and ducts of the testes.

Connective tissues

Connective tissues, as the name implies, connect the various cells of other tissues and organs and their function is largely mechanical. They include the following tissues: (1) areolar, (2) elastic, (3) lymphatic or reticular, (4) adipose, (5) fibrous, (6) cartilaginous and (7) bony.

(1) *Areolar tissue* is composed of white and elastic fibres forming meshworks that enclose spaces or *areolae*, e.g. *subcutaneous tissue*.

(2) *Elastic tissue* is composed of yellow elastic fibres. It is found in the walls of blood vessels, the lungs and most characteristically in the *ligamentum nuchae*.

(3) *Lymphatic* or *reticular tissue* is composed of networks of collagenous fibres enclosing *lymph*.

(4) *Adipose tissue* or *fat* is composed of a network in which are embedded *fat cells*. The chief constituents of animal fat are *stearin, olein* and *plamitin*. The body fat comes partly from fat in the diet and is in part manufactured, within the body, from carbohydrates and sometimes proteins in the diet.

  The fat is soft during life but quickly hardens after death. This is due to the fall in temperature and not to *rigor mortis*. Fat is found under the skin, the *subcutaneous fat* or *panniculus adiposus*, and collects around the heart and particularly around the kidneys. It is also found in the pleura, peritoneum and mesentery and in small quantities in the tissues of most organs. Fat provides a store of energy for the body. Being a poor conductor of heat it prevents loss of body heat. In well-fed animals it is found between the muscle fibres and is called *marbling*.

  Unlike ruminants, horses and pigs tend to deposit fat unchanged. Fat varies in consistency, colour and distribution (Table 1.1). Some animals have white fat and some yellow due to the presence of *carotene*. In some the fat is firm, in others soft. In chronic diseases the fat may not set and remains soft. The colour may vary not only with the species but also with the age and breed of the animal.

  In old cows the fat is yellow. The Channel Island breeds of cattle have a yellow fat although young calves of those breeds have white fat. The colour

Table 1.1 Characteristics of fat.

Animal	Colour	Consistency
Calf	White or greyish white	Soft and gelatinous
Heifer and bullock	White or yellowish white	Firm and smooth
Cow	Yellow	Fairly firm and ragged
Bull	White or yellowish white	Firm (sparse)
Sheep and goat	Very white	Very firm and crisp
Pig	White	Fairly firm and greasy
Horse	Yellowish white	Soft and greasy
Deer	White	Firm (very sparse)

may also vary with the feeding, e.g. a grass diet with high levels of carotene gives a yellow fat compared to the white fat in barley beef.

The consistency of fat varies according to the amounts of stearin, olein and palmitin in it. A high stearin content gives a firm consistency, whilst a high olein content gives an oily consistency. A good knowledge of the different kinds of fat is very helpful in identifying the source of specimens.

Brown fat is a type of fat, deposits of which are found scattered throughout the body, mainly in the neck and axillary regions. It has a richer blood supply than normal fat, and can be converted more easily into energy. Therefore it has the ability to keep animals lean. Lean animals have more brown fat than fat animals.

(5) *Fibrous tissue* is composed almost entirely of white fibres. It is found in ligaments, tendons and fasciae and in the serous membranes.

(6) *Cartilaginous tissue* (cartilage), commonly known as gristle, is a specialised dense connective tissue. It forms most of the temporary skeleton of the mammalian embryo and persists in the adult, e.g. at the joint surfaces, in the respiratory passages, in the ears, and as the costal cartilages of the ribs. The commonest and most characteristic form of cartilage is known as *hyaline cartilage* because of its glassy translucent appearance. Cartilage in some areas, e.g. at the pelvic symphysis and at the dorsal extremities of the spines of the first five or six thoracic vertebrae, gradually ossifies with age. It is therefore helpful in deciding upon the age of an animal.

(7) *Bony tissue.* Bone is a connective tissue that is impregnated with salts of lime, chiefly phosphate, these salts constituting about two-thirds the weight of the bone.

Bony tissue is either *compact* or *spongy*. Compact bone is white, dense and almost like ivory. Spongy bone consists of delicate bony plates and spicules that run in various directions and intercross. The spaces between the plates are called *marrow spaces* and are filled with *marrow*. Externally, bones are covered, except at the joints, by a vascular, fibrous membrane – the *periosteum* (Fig. 1.2).

The bones are commonly divided into four classes:

(i)   Long bones – typically elongated cylindrical form with enlarged extremities, e.g. femur.

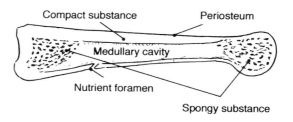

Fig. 1.2 Long bone.

(ii)   Flat bones – bones of the skull.

(iii)   Short bones – e.g. those of carpus and tarsus, with somewhat similar dimensions in length, breadth and thickness. They diminish friction or change directions of tendons.

(iv)   Irregular bones – bones of irregular shape, e.g. vertebrae.

Marrow

There are two distinct varieties of marrow – the red marrow and the yellow marrow.

(1)   The red marrow occupies the spaces in the spongy bone; it is highly vascular and thus maintains the nutrition of the spongy bone. It is in these situations that the red blood corpuscles are formed.

(2)   The yellow marrow fills the medullary cavity of long bones and consists chiefly of fat cells with numerous blood vessels.

NB In young animals there is only red marrow, i.e. as the animal ages the proportion of red to yellow decreases.

Short descriptions of the muscular and lymphatic tissues are given in the relevant chapters.

Chapter 2
Deer and Venison

Deer are ruminants related to cattle and sheep. Venison, or deer meat, is becoming increasingly important both for home consumption and for export.

Six species of deer are found wild in Britain: red, roe, fallow, sika, muntjac and Chinese water deer. Two other species, wapiti and Père David's, are found in deer farms, deer parks and zoos. Wapiti are used for experimental cross-breeding purposes. Red deer and roe deer account for about 80% of the venison produced. Red deer is by far the most important species both in the wild and in deer farms. There are over 300 000 red deer in the Highlands of Scotland alone, and the 40 000 wild red deer shot every year, plus several thousand roe deer, provide the raw material for the Scottish game industry.

Deer killed in the wild are shot by sportsmen or stalkers. Sportsmen do not aim for the head because it is generally wanted as a trophy and many deer are therefore shot through the chest or abdomen. This results in considerable damage and contamination, and much meat is rejected as unfit for human consumption. Deer should be gralloched (entrails removed) as quickly as possible to delay the onset of putrefaction. The entrails are generally discarded on the hills.

The regulations require that the red offal, i.e. the lungs, heart, liver and kidneys, be retained for inspection and that they be identifiable with the carcass. The carcass is collected, having discarded the remaining offal, and hung in a properly constructed larder. The pelvis and sternum are split open and the inside of the carcass is washed out with clean water. The carcass is kept propped open with a metal spreader. When cool, the red offal is kept identifiable with the carcass. The stalker is required to report any abnormality seen in the 'green' offal left on the hills. The carcass has to be removed to the game factory in a refrigerated van with hanging rails and it must be kept in skin.

The carcass and offal are examined by a Local Veterinary Inspector (LVI (meat)). The carcass is examined for:

(1) General state of nutrition
(2) Evidence of disease
(3) Contamination.

The lungs are palpated, and the mediastinal and bronchial nodes and liver and heart are incised.

Farmed deer come under the Fresh Meat (Hygiene and Inspection) Regulations 1995 and can be slaughtered in a slaughterhouse or farmed game handling facility. Inspection is carried out by inspectors of the Meat Hygiene Service in these licensed premises.

Table 2.1 shows the terms used when referring to the various species of deer. All the males (except the male Chinese water deer) have antlers, which are cast each year. None of the females has antlers.

Table 2.1   Terms and data concerning deer.

Species	Male	Antlers cast	Female	Young	Gestation period (days)
Red	Stag	Mar–April	Hind	Calf	231
Fallow	Buck	April–May	Doe	Fawn	234
Sika	Stag	Mar–April	Hind	Calf	220
Roe	Buck	Oct–Dec	Doe	Kid	294*
Muntjac	Buck	May–June	Doe	Fawn	210
Chinese water	Buck	No antlers	Doe	Fawn	176
Wapiti	Bull	Feb–March	Cow	Calf	250
Père David's	Stag	Oct	Hind	Calf	280

The species are listed in descending order of size.
* This includes 5 months' delayed implantation.

The young are born between late May and the end of June and are spotted when born.

Close seasons are imposed by law to protect deer during the rut, calving and early rearing periods. During the 2–5 week period of the rut the male ceases to eat and may lose a quarter of his body weight. The close seasons are as shown in Table 2.2.

Table 2.2   Deer close seasons in England and Scotland.

Species	Male	Female
England		
Red	1 May–31 July	1 May–31 Oct
Fallow	1 May–31 July	1 May–31 Oct
Sika	1 May–31 July	1 May–31 Oct
Roe	1 May–31 July	1 May–31 Oct
Scotland		
Red	21 Oct–30 June	16 Feb–20 Oct
Fallow	1 May–31 July	16 Feb–20 Oct
Sika	1 May–31 July	16 Feb–20 Oct
Roe	21 Oct–31 July	1 Mar–20 Oct

Venison is a very lean meat and there is no marbling. the fat content is approximately 5%, which is almost exactly a quarter of that of beef, lamb and pork. Also, 50% of deer fat is polyunsaturated compared with 4–5% in cattle, sheep and pig.

Deer have a larger mass of skeletal muscle associated with their legs, especially the hind legs, in comparison with sheep, cattle and pigs.

The quality of venison sold to the public varies greatly and much more than that of any other meat. This is due to the varying conditions, e.g. age, amount of food available, rearing conditions, and the treatment of the carcasses thereafter.

Venison from adult males killed during the rutting season may have a strong odour.

The body weight of deer depends greatly on the climate and abundance of food, e.g. a large red deer stag reared in the south of England can weigh as much as 180 kg (400 lb) as against 130 kg (280 lb) for a stag in the Highlands of Scotland.

The best venison is that of deer between 8 months and 2 years 6 months of age.

Some reindeer are slaughtered for human consumption in this country. The carcass is not so well muscled as the red deer carcass.

Anatomy and diseases of deer are dealt with in the relevant chapters.

Venison as food has only fairly recently become important. Therefore information on diseases and post-mortem findings of deer is relatively sparse, unlike that on cattle, sheep and pigs. This will rapidly change as more people become involved. Deer in the wild are relatively free from disease, but as farming of deer becomes more intensive it is almost inevitable that many diseases will become increasingly common.

Systems of the Body

For ease of description the systems of the body have been grouped under nine headings: skeletal, muscular, circulatory, lymphatic, respiratory, digestive, urogenital, nervous and endocrine. The information on these systems is very basic and is almost entirely concerned with identification purposes. Fuller information should be obtained from anatomy textbooks.

Chapter 3
Skeletal System

The skeletal system consists of a framework composed of the bones of the body. These are joined together in their natural positions by ligaments and joints. The softer tissues of the body are built on this framework and the organs are enclosed and partly protected by it.

Bones

The skull and lower jaw

The upper jaw is attached to the skull and contains the upper teeth. The lower jaw or mandible, carrying the lower teeth, is a separate bone joined to the skull by means of ligaments. The skull articulates with the first cervical vertebra, the atlas, by a ball-and-socket joint.

The vertebral column

The vertebral column, spine or backbone consists of many vertebrae, which form a long, fairly flexible chain extending from the head to the tail. The vertebrae are divided into groups named according to their position:

(1) Cervical (C) or neck vertebrae.
(2) Dorsal or thoracic (T) vertebrae – those of the back with which the ribs articulate.
(3) Lumbar (L) vertebrae – situated in the region of the loin.
(4) Sacral (S) vertebrae – in the pelvic region. These are generally fused together to form the sacrum and articulate with the pelvic bones to form the pelvis.
(5) Coccygeal (Cy) or tail vertebrae.

The vertebral formulae for the various animals are shown in Table 3.1. From this it will be noted that they all have seven cervical vertebrae. Even the giraffe with its very long neck has the same number.

The spinal cord passes through the vertebral foramen of each vertebra down to

Table 3.1   Vertebral formulae.

	C	T	L	S	Cy
Horse	7	18	6	5	15–21
Ox	7	13	6	5	18–20
Deer	7	13	6–7	4	10
Sheep	7	13	6–7	4	16–18
Pig	7	14–15	6–7	4	20–23

about the third sacral vertebra. Between the bodies of the vertebrae (except in the sacral region where they are fused together) are found elastic cartilaginous pads or *intervertebral discs*. (See Figs 3.1 and 3.2.)

The ribs

These are long curved paired bones that help to form the sides of the chest wall. They are attached above on each side to the dorsal or thoracic vertebrae (same number) and below to the sternum, or to one another. The ribs that articulate with the sternum are known as true ribs, while those that fail to reach the sternum articulate with erach other and are known as false ribs. The ribs are separated from one another by spaces, the intercostal spaces containing muscle tissue (the intercostal muscles).

The sternum

The sternum or breast bone is a long bone made up of 6–8 segments joined together by cartilage. The superior surface is concave and forms part of the floor of the thorax.

The sacrum

The sacrum is formed by the fusion of the sacral vertebrae and is commonly described as one bone. It is traingular in outline, articulates very firmly on each side and is wedged between the ilia.

The os coxae (pelvic bones) (Fig. 3.3)

Each os coxae, right and left, consists of the following three bones, which fuse together to form one large flat bone:

(1)   The *ilium* is the largest of the three. It articulates with the sacrum.
(2)   The *ischium* is the most posterior and forms the posterior part of the floor of the pelvis.
(3)   The *pubis* is the smallest of the three bones and forms the anterior floor of the pelvis.

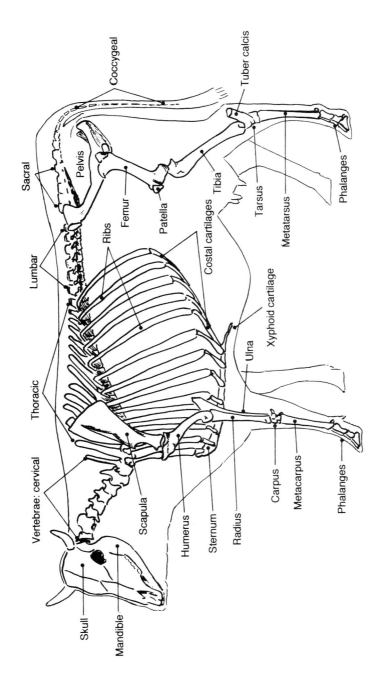

Fig. 3.1   Skeleton of cow.

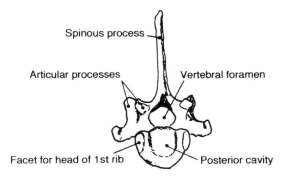

Fig. 3.2   The 7th cervical vertebra of ox.

All three bones join to form the *acetabulum* into which the head of the femur fits.

The ischium and pubis join with their opposite bones at the *symphysis pelvis*, the anterior part of which is the *symphysis pubis*.

The body cavities

(1)   The cranial cavity is the cavity formed by the bones of the skull. It contains the brain.

(2)   The *thorax* or thoracic cavity is formed by the thoracic vertebrae above, the ribs at the sides and the sternum below. It is cone-shaped and is separated from the abdominal cavity by a strong muscular membrane, the *diaphragm*. The thorax contains part of the oesophagus, part of the trachea or windpipe, the heart, the lungs, part of the thymus gland and portions of the great blood vessels.

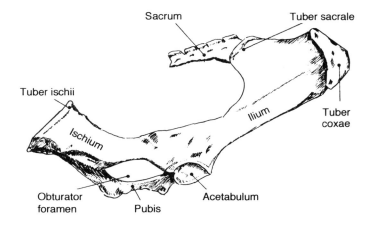

Fig. 3.3   Right pelvic bones of ox.

(3) The *abdomen* or abdominal cavity is formed by the lumbar vertebrae above, while the abdominal muscles form its sides and lower wall. The front wall is formed by the diaphragm. The abdomen contains the stomach, intestines, liver, spleen, pacreas, kidneys and bladder when it is extended, and the uterus in the pregnant female.

(4) The *pelvis* or pelvic cavity is formed by the sacrum above and the pelvic bones on either side and below. It contains the rectum, the bladder and, in the non-pregnant or newly-pregnant female, the uterus and ovaries.

The bones of the fore limb *(Fig. 3.1)*

(1) The *scapula* or shoulder blade is a flat triangular bone which has no articulation with the chest wall but is attached to it by muscles.

(2) The *humerus* is a long cylindrical bone that extends from the shoulder to the elbow joint.

(3) The *radius* and *ulna*. The radius is the larger bone and extends from the elbow to the knee joint. The ulna in cattle is fused to the radius. Its upper end forms a projection known as the olecranon process or 'point of the elbow'.

(4) The *carpus* or knee joint is made up of six small bones disposed in two rows. The upper row articulates with the radius, the lower with the metacarpus.

(5) The *metacarpus* or cannon bone is a cylindrical bone that extends from the knee joint to the digits.

(6) The *digits*, or bones of the foot. In the ox there are two digits separated by a cleft ('cloven footed'). Each digit is composed of three phalanges. The terminal portion of each digit is surrounded by the hoof.

(7) the *navicular* bone is a small bone at the back of the last joint.

The bones of the hind limb *(Fig. 3.1)*

(1) The *femur* or thigh bone is a large, strong, cylindrical bone that extends from the hip joint above to the stifle below. The upper rounded head fits into the socket or acetabulum in the os coxae to which it is attached by the *round ligament*. The lower end articulates with the tibia, fibula and patella or kneecap.

(2) The *patella* or kneecap is a small flat bone roughly triangular with the apex below. It articulates with the femur and is attached to the tibia by means of three strong fibrous bands or ligaments.

(3) The *tibia* and *fibula* or leg bones articulate above with the femur and below with the tarsal bones, i.e. they extend from the stifle to the tarsus. The fibula is rudimentary in ruminants.

(4) The *tarsus* or hock, like the carpus, consists of two rows of small bones. The upper row contains two segments, the posterior of which – the os calcis – has a marked projection, the 'point of the hock'. The lower row has three bones.

(5)   The *metatarsus* extends from the hock to the fetlock and is similar to but slightly longer than the metacarpus in the fore limb.
(6)   The *digits* are the same as in the fore limb.

Differential features of bones

The following are some of the distinctions between bones of the various animals.

Horse and ox *(Fig. 3.4)*

(1)   The spinal processes of the anterior dorsal vertebrae of the horse are shorter and stouter.
(2)   The ribs of the ox are smoother and in the lower two-thirds are broader. The ox has 13 pairs of ribs whereas the horse has 18 pairs.
(3)   The scapula of the ox is more regularly triangular than that of the horse and the spine is more prominent and placed further forward, so that the supraspinous fossa, i.e. the part in front of the spine, is narrow and does not extend to the lower part of the bone. Instead of subsiding as in the horse, the spine rises and had a pointed projection – the acromion. There is a distinct notch in the glenoid cavity of the horse, but not in that of the ox. The glenoid cavity is the articular surface of the scapula.
(4)   The humerus of the horse has three tuberosities, i.e. the lateral tuberosity is divided in two giving a bicipital groove. In the ox the lateral tuberosity is very large and rises 2.5–5 cm above the level of the bone.
(5)   The ulna extends only half way down the radius in the horse. In the ox it is more developed and reaches the carpus.
(6)   The small head of the fibula in the ox is hook-shaped. In the horse it is separate and extends two-thirds down the tibia.

Sheep, goat and deer

(1)   The bones of the goat and deer are more slender and longer than those of the sheep, and the bony processes are longer and more sharply edged than in the sheep.
(2)   The scapula of the sheep is shorter compared with its breadth and the edge of the spine in the centre is thickened backwards, while in the goat and deer it is straight and unthickened.

Cat and rabbit *(Figs 3.5 and 3.6)*

(1)   The lateral processes of the lumbar vertebrae in the cat are pointed whereas in the rabbit there are two extensions, one backwards and one forwards

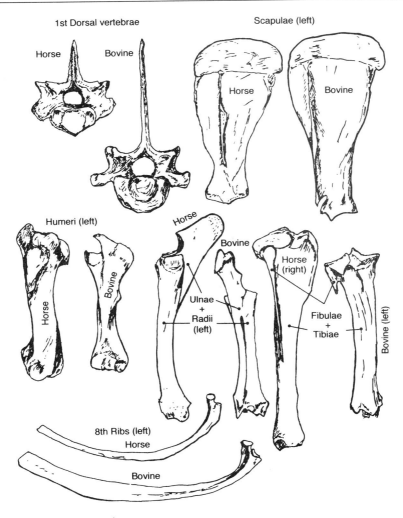

Fig. 3.4 Bones of horse and ox.

(2) In the cat there are 13 pairs of rounded ribs, whilst in the rabbit there are 12 pairs which are more flat.

(3) The rabbit has a long metacromion on the scapula directed backwards, which is absent in the cat.

(4) The tibia and fibula in the cat are separate for their complete length. In the rabbit they are separate only in the upper half.

(5) The radius and ulna are separate in the cat but united in the rabbit.

(6) The male cat has an os penis.

(7) The coccygeal vertebrae in the rabbit are very small.

Cat bones are included because of complaints from members of the public that they have been served cat meat instead of rabbit or chicken in oriental restaurants.

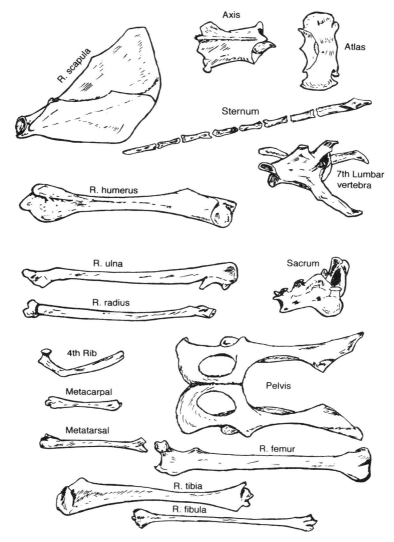

Fig. 3.5 Bones of cat.

Fowl and rabbit *(Figs 3.6, 3.7 and 23.4)*

(1) The bones of fowl tend to be whiter in colour and larger in all dimensions than the rabbit.

(2) The humerus is hollow in fowl.

(3) The metatarsus is very large in fowl and has a spur in the male.

(4) The ribs are flat with uncinate processes projecting backwards in fowl. In the rabbit the ribs are long and slender with no uncinate processes.

(5) In fowl the pelvis and sternum are very typical and not at all like those in mammals.

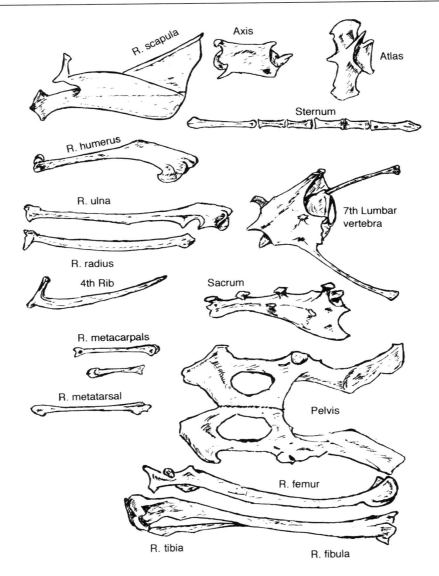

Fig. 3.6   Bones of rabbit.

(6) In fowl the clavicle (wishbone) is present as also is the coracoid, but these are absent in the rabbit.

(7) The fowl scapula is not the typical triangular shape.

(8) The sternal bones are fused in fowl, but not in the rabbit.

(9) The pygostyle is present in fowl.

In food inspection departments it is very useful to have skeletons of the various animals. This is of course difficult with the large animals because of the space

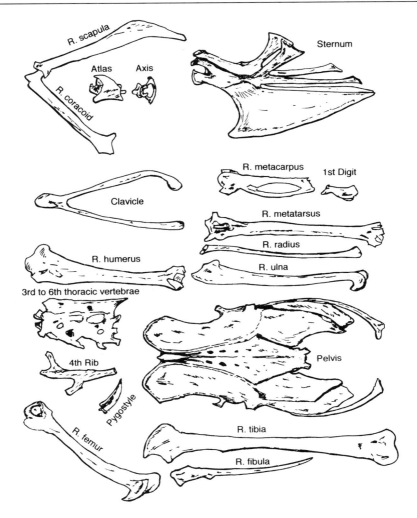

Fig. 3.7   Bones of fowl.

they occupy. However, with the small animals, e.g. rabbit, fowl and duck, it is quite simple to mount their bones on thick plastic sheets.

This makes it much easier to identify bones, the origin of which may be in question.

Joints

An articulation or joint is formed by the union of two or more bones or cartilage by other tissue. Bone is the fundamental part of most joints; in some cases a bone and a cartilage, or two cartilages, form a joint.

Joints are classified in various ways but the simplest way is as follows.

(1) *Immovable joints*, e.g. those of the skull and pelvis. The bones of the skull are united by means of irregular saw-like edges known as sutures, which firmly bind them together without intervention of cartilage.
(2) *Slightly movable joints*. In this type of joint the opposed bony surfaces are covered by hyaline cartilage and connected by a fibro-cartilaginous pad. Two examples are joints between the bodies of vertebrae and the joint between the two pubic bones in young animals.
(3) *Movable joints* (Fig. 3.8). These are made up of the following tissues:

    (a) Cartilage, known as articular cartilage, covers the surface of the part of the bone that enters into the joint.
    (b) The capsule, which consists of strong fibrous tissue, is attached to the rim of the articular cartilage. The capsule encloses the joint cavity.
    (c) The synovial membrane. This is composed of endothelial cells, and lines the inside of the joint cavity. It secretes an oily liquid, *synovial fluid*, which facilitates smooth movement.
    (d) Blood vessels, lymph vessels and nerves supply the joint.

Movable joints are further classified by their type of movement:

(1) Ball-and-socket joint, e.g. the hip joint.
(2) Gliding joint, e.g. the joints between the articular processes of the vertebrae.
(3) Hinge joint, which allows movement in one plane, e.g. the elbow joint.
(4) Condyloid joint, which allows movement in two planes, e.g. the joint between skull and lower jaw.
(5) Pivot joint, which allows rotation, e.g. the atlanto-axial joint.

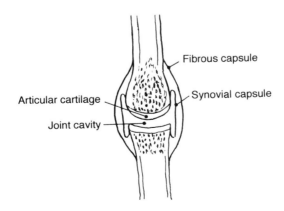

Fig. 3.8 Simple joint.

Ligaments

These are usually composed of strong bands of white fibrous tissue that bind the bones together. They are very pliable but not elastic. An exception to this is the *ligamentum nuchae*, which is composed of yellow elastic tissue. It is a very strong ligament that extends from the occipital bone to the top of the spines of the thoracic vertebrae where it is continuous with the *supraspinous ligament*.

Chapter 4
Muscular System

The movements of animals are brought about by the contraction of muscles. The muscles contract or shorten in response to impulses conveyed to them by nerves. Muscles only stretch beyond the normal in abnormal situations resulting in strains or torn muscles. Most are attached to bones which, with joints, act as levers and hinges. For convenience the term *origin* is used for the attachment that remains stationary when the muscle contracts, whereas the movable attachment is called the *insertion*.

Muscle tissue is composed of small elongated cells or *muscle fibres*. These are bound in *bundles* by connective tissue. The fibres vary much in size but average 2.5 cm × 0.05 mm. They are cylindrical in shape with rounded ends. Many become elongated into *tendons*, which attach or insert into bones. The fibres consist of a sheath or *sarcolemma* enclosing the *contractile substance*.

There are three types of muscles:

(1) *Voluntary, skeletal* or *cross-striated muscles*, which are under the control of the will. They constitute the muscular apparatus attached to the bones and are commonly called meat or flesh.

(2) *Cardiac* or *heart muscle* is also striated but otherwise different from voluntary muscle. It is not under the control of the will but, like the involuntary muscles, is controlled by the autonomic nervous system.

(3) *Involuntary, plain* or *non-striated muscles* are not under the control of the will, e.g. the muscular layer of the intestinal wall.

Again it is emphasised that detailed information on the muscular system should be obtained from textbooks on anatomy.

Chapter 5
Circulatory System

The circulatory system consists of the blood and the means by which it is circulated round the body, i.e. the heart, arteries, veins and capillaries.

The *blood* is concerned with external and internal respiration, i.e. in the lungs and in the tissues. Together with the lymph it is the transport medium of the body. The arterial blood, which is bright red, carries nutrients and oxygen to the tissues. The venous blood is dark red and carries waste products, including carbon dioxide, away from the tissues.

Blood consists of a yellowish fluid called *plasma* in which the blood cells are suspended. There are three main types of blood cells:

(1) *Red blood corpuscles* or *erythrocytes*, which are made in the bone marrow
(2) *White blood corpuscles* or *leucocytes*, which are made in the bone marrow, spleen and lymph nodes
(3) *Platelets*.

The erythrocytes have no nuclei in mammals but are nucleated in birds. The leucocytes are nucleated. In mammals there are 7 000 000–10 000 000 erythrocytes per cubic millimetre of blood and 8000–20 000 leucocytes.

Blood normally remains fluid in the blood vessels during life but rapidly clots when shed. Clotting is due to the formation of a jelly by the deposition of an insoluble protein called *fibrin*. Calcium, which is a normal constituent of the blood, is necessary for clotting. If blood is collected and citrate added immediately, clotting does not occur. This is because the calcium is taken out of solution. Practical use is made of this fact when blood is collected for making black puddings.

Clotting can also be prevented by adding *heparin* or by stirring vigorously, when the fibrin can be removed as a white stringy material. Plasma with the fibrin and blood cells removed is called *serum*. Clotting can be shown as a series of reactions:

(1) Injured tissue cells + platelets → *thrombokinase*
(2) *Thrombokinase + prothrombin* + calcium → *thrombin*
(3) *Thrombin + Fibrinogen* → *Fibrin* (insoluble clot). The fibrin entangles the corpuscles forming the clot.

The heart (Fig. 5.1) is the muscular pump of the circulatory system (Fig. 5.2). It lies in the thoracic cavity between the right and left lungs and is enclosed in a fibro-serous sac called the *pericardium*. This is relatively thin but strong and inelastic. It is smooth and glistening and contains a small amount of *pericardial fluid*. Like other serous membranes it is regarded as consisting of a *parietal* and a *visceral* part. The parietal part lines the fibrous part to which it is closely attached. The visceral part covers the heart and part of the large blood vessels and is called the *epicardium*.

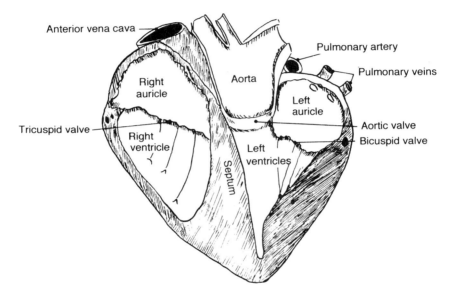

Fig. 5.1 Heart.

The interior of the heart is divided by a longitudinal partition or *septum* into two muscular cavities, the right and left. Each of the chambers is again divided transversely into upper and lower portions called the *auricle* and *ventricle*. Thus there are four chambers in the heart: right auricle, right ventricle, left auricle and left ventricle. The *tricuspid valve* is the valve between the right auricle and ventricle and the one between the left auricle and ventricle is the *bicuspid valve*.

The left ventricle is very muscular and thus thick-walled, because it has to pump the blood throughout the body. The right ventricle is thin walled as it only has to pump the blood through the lungs.

On the external surface there are various furrows or grooves, which are a help in identification. The coronary furrow indicates the division between the auricles and ventricles. It almost completely encircles the heart except at the origin of the pulmonary artery. The right and left ventricular furrows correspond to the septum between the ventricles. They commence at the coronary

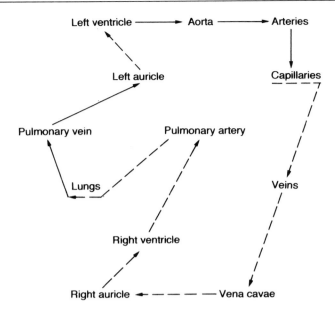

Fig. 5.2 Circulation of the blood. **NB** The pulmonary vein carries *arterial* blood and the pulmonary artery carries *venous* blood.

furrow and run at right angles to it towards the apex of the heart. The furrows are occupied by the coronary blood vessels (the blood vessels of the heart itself) and by fat.

Arteries, *veins* and *capillaries*, the blood vessels, carry the blood around the body to and from the tissues and organs. They consist of a completely closed system.

The arteries are thick-walled and consist of three layers: an inner or elastic layer lined by *endothelium*, a middle or muscular layer and an outer or areolar layer.

The veins resemble the arteries but contain less elastic and muscular tissues and are therefore thinner walled. Many of the larger veins have valves that prevent back-flow of blood.

The capillaries are the smallest blood vessels. The arterial and venous capillaries join together forming networks.

The smaller the blood vessels become, the fewer muscular and elastic tissues they have. The finest capillaries are composed only of tubes of flattened endothelial cells. It is here that the exchange of materials takes place between the blood, the tissue fluid and the body cells. The arterial blood brings oxygen and other nutrients to the cells. The venous capillaries take away the waste products, i.e. most of the carbon dioxide. The rest, which is of bigger particle size, is taken away by the lymph capillaries. It is important to remember that oxygen and carbon dioxide are not transported free in the blood but each is bound to blood proteins, the chief of which is haemoglobin.

Ox heart *(Fig. 5.3)*

(1)   There are three ventricular furrows:

    (a)   The right or posterior furrow extends to about 3–4 cm above the apex.

    (b)   The left or anterior furrow runs almost parallel to the posterior border and ends at the apex. There is much more fat at the coronary furrow end of the left furrow than at the corresponding ends of the other two ventricular furrows.

    (c)   The intermediate furrow is shallow and extends down the left side of the posterior border but does not reach the apex.

(2)   Two bones (*ossa cordis*) are present in the aortic ring (a fibrous ring at the origin of the aorta). The right one is irregularly triangular in shape. The left bone is smaller and inconstant.

(3)   The weight is 2 kg approximately.

(4)   The ox heart is relatively longer than the horse heart and the base is smaller.

(5)   The ventricular part is more conical and more pointed than the horse heart.

(6)   The amount of fat in or near the furrows is much greater than in the horse. The fat is also firmer and not so yellow.

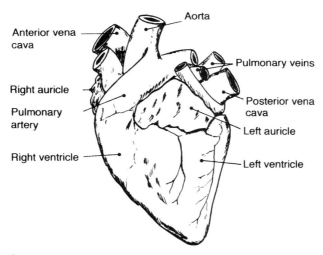

Fig. 5.3   Heart of ox.

Sheep heart (similar to ox)

(1)   Firm, white fat is present on the upper portion.

(2)   The *ossa cordis* are generally absent but may be present in old sheep.

(3)   The breadth at the base usually equals the length.

(4)   The weight is 100 g approximately.

(5)   The sheep heart is relatively smaller and more pointed than the calf heart, and the pulmonary artery has a much smaller diameter and a thinner wall.

Goat heart (similar to sheep)

Pig heart (Fig. 5.4)

(1) The pig heart is more globular than the sheep and calf hearts, being broad and short with a blunt apex.
(2) The fat is soft and greasy.
(3) The heart looks twisted as the right ventricle appears to sag.
(4) There are either two or three ventricular furrows:

  (a) The right furrow runs obliquely across the heart.
  (b) The left furrow is almost parallel with the left border.
  (c) An intermediate furrow may be present or absent. When present it is small and situated on the left border, and may extend to the apex.

(5) The lower edge of the left auricle is notched and lower than the right one.
(6) The weight obviously varies greatly according to the size of the pig. In a pig of 100 kg dressed weight, the heart weighs approximately 250 g.

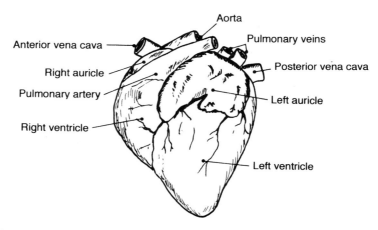

Fig. 5.4 Heart of pig.

Horse heart (Fig. 5.5)

(1) There are two ventricular furrows:

  (a) The right furrow begins at the coronary furrow just below the posterior vena cava and ends about 3–4 cm above the apex.
  (b) The left furrow descends almost parallel to the posterior border and ends at the apex.

(2) There are no *ossa cordis*.
(3) The horse heart is less elongated than the ox heart and has a bigger base.
(4) There is less fat than on the ox heart and it is oily and yellow.
(5) Weight variable.

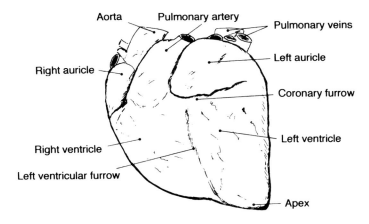

Fig. 5.5 Heart of horse.

Deer heart *(Fig. 5.6)*

(1) There are three ventricular furrows and although there is very little fat present the coronary blood vessels show up very clearly.
(2) The auricles are situated very high up on the heart.
(3) The heart is relatively bigger than that of the sheep and the cardiac muscle is very firm.
(4) There is very little fat in the coronary and ventricular furrows.

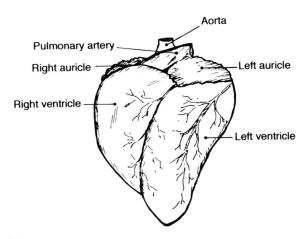

Fig. 5.6 Heart of deer.

The fetal circulation (Fig. 5.7)

The fetus has no independent respiration or digestion and therefore depends entirely on the oxygen and nutritive substances that diffuse through the cotyledons from the mother's blood. It must be understood that there is no direct

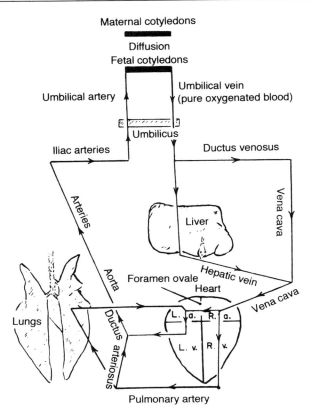

Fig. 5.7 Fetal circulation.

connection between the maternal and fetal circulations, i.e. the blood of the mother and the blood of the fetus do not normally mix.

The oxygenated blood flowing from the fetal cotyledons through the umbilical vein is partly conveyed to the posterior vena cava by means of the *ductus venosus*. However, the greater quantity of the blood mixes, within the liver, with the portal stream returning blood from the intestine. From the liver it is conveyed to the vena cava by the hepatic veins.

When blood reaches the right auricle, most of it passes through an opening, the *foramen ovale* (foramen means a small opening, from the Latin *forare*, to pierce) to the left auricle. Some, however, passes into the right ventricle from which it is transported by the pulmonary artery. This blood is again divided, some going to the lungs for their nutrition, but most goes via the *ductus arteriosus* to the aorta.

From the left auricle the blood passes into the left ventricle to be pumped via the aorta to all the arteries of the fetal body. The blood reaching the iliac arteries passes to the umbilical artery at the umbilicus. From there it goes to the fetal cotyledons to be reoxygenated, etc. and thence to the umbilical veins.

After birth the *foramen ovale* soon closes. The *ductus venosus, ductus arteriosus* and the umbilical vessels become impervious cords.

Chapter 6
Lymphatic System

In animals the blood vessels form a completely closed system in which the very thin-walled blood capillaries are the most numerous vessels. Oxygen and nutrient materials pass into the tissue fluid through the capillary walls that surround the tissue cells, and which are in close contact with them. The cells take up these materials in exchange for carbon dioxide and waste products. Most of the carbon dioxide is taken away by the venous capillaries. The remainder and the larger particle-sized waste products are taken up by the lymph capillaries.

The lymphatics begin as a network of very fine lymph capillaries with blind extremities. Like the blood capillaries they are separated from the tissue fluid by a thin layer of endothelial cells. The lymphatic capillaries gradually enlarge into thin-walled vessels, the lymphatic vessels. These are similar to veins but are finer and have more valves. Even the largest lymphatic vessels are very small and are difficult to see with the naked eye. When filled with fluid – the *lymph* – they have a characteristic beaded appearance.

The propulsion of lymph is partly due to slight tissue pressure, which helps to drive fluid from the tissue spaces into the lymphatic capillaries. However, the main factor in the propulsion is the normal muscular movements of the animal.

Lymph is generally colourless or yellowish. It is similar to blood plasma but is not so rich in protein, and is thinner and more watery. Practically all the lymph vessels discharge the lymph into lymph nodes before it goes back into the blood stream. The lymph nodes play an important part in filtering out bacteria, foreign substances, etc.

Lymphatic vessels that convey lymph to and from a lymph node are known as *afferent lymphatics* and *efferent lymphatics*, respectively. Areas drained by lymph nodes are known as *drainage areas*. A knowledge of the positions of lymph nodes and their drainage areas is of the greatest importance in meat inspection.

After lymph has passed through one or more lymph nodes it is carried by efferent vessels to larger lymph vessels. The largest of these is the *thoracic duct*, which opens into the anterior vena cava. It collects lymph from the posterior part of the body and the intestines. Lymph from the anterior part of the body is collected by two *tracheal lymph ducts*, which discharge into the *jugular veins* and *thoracic duct* (Fig. 6.1).

The lymphatic vessels of the intestinal canal are called *lacteals* because during

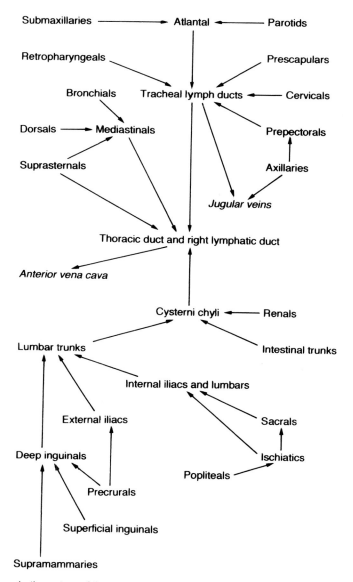

Fig. 6.1 Lymphatic system of the ox.

digestion (if the meal contains fat) the fluid contained in them resembles milk in appearance. The lymph during the period of digestion is called *chyle*. Chyle is lymph containing finely divided fat globules.

The cavities of the serous membranes, i.e. the pleura and peritoneum, are part of the lymphatic system. They are moistened with lymph and are in communication with lymphatic vessels. The spleen is also part of the lymphatic system.

Lymph nodes (Fig. 6.2)

An intimate knowledge of the normal condition and position of the lymph nodes and of their drainage areas is of the greatest importance in meat inspection. Swollen and haemorrhagic lymph nodes are an indication of abnormal conditions in the animal body – disease, bruising, etc. On incision of the nodes, various types of lesions may be found, e.g. those of tuberculosis, actinobacillosis, etc.

The size of the lymph nodes varies from that of a pin head to 10–20 cm or more. In the horse, the nodes are small and occur in large numbers, forming grape-like groups, whilst in ruminants they consist of a few glands of large size only. In older animals the nodes are smaller than in younger animals. The nodes are generally round or oval in form and somewhat pressed together. On incision a small quantity of lymph exudes. In consistency the nodes are firm, rather than soft, and in colour may be white, grey or greyish-blue. The lymph vessels are seldom visible to the naked eye. Small, dark red nodes, *haemal lymph nodes*, are often found in association with lymph nodes. They are said to be small accessory spleens. They are common in sheep, especially in the lumbar and pelvic regions in association with the lymph nodes. Because of their dark red colour they are easily seen. They are not so common in pigs and are absent or very rare in cattle and horses.

Principal lymph nodes of cattle

Lymph nodes are nearly always embedded in fat and therefore are not easily seen without incision.

Students should take every opportunity to incise lymph nodes as this is the only way of becoming familiar with their positions in the offal and carcass.

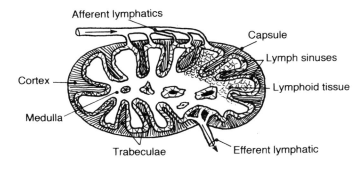

Fig. 6.2   Section of lymph node.

Head

Retropharyngeal (one each side)

Located on the side and posterior to the pharynx near to the attachments of the cornua of the hyoid bone to the skull. It is relatively large, and afferent vessels come from the tongue, floor of the mouth, hard and soft palate, gums, pharynx, submaxillary salivary glands, posterior part of nasal cavity, base of skull and the larynx. The efferent vessels help to form the tracheal lymph ducts.

Submaxillary (one each side)

This is superficial on the inner side of the lower jaw near its angle, about 5 cm anterior to the point at which the lower jaw curves upwards. The afferent vessels come from the muzzle, lips, cheeks, hard palate, anterior part of the turbinate bones and nasal septum, part of the gums, salivary glands, tip of the tongue and the anterior muscles of the head. The efferent vessels go to the atlantal node, which is unimportant in meat inspection.

Parotid (one each side)

Located on the edge of the masseter muscle and covered by the parotid salivary gland, which has to be incised to expose it – about 3 cm in front of the ear and a little lower than the external meatus. The afferent vessels come from the muzzle, lips, gums in part, the anterior part of the turbinates and nasal septum, the parotid salivary gland, most of the head muscles, and the bones and skin of the head. The efferent vessels go to the atlantal node.

Lungs

Left bronchial

This lies under the aortic arch and on the origin of the left bronchus.

Right bronchial

It is smaller than the left bronchial and lies on the origin of the right bronchus.

Mediastinals

These are a chain of fairly large lymph nodes, which lie in the mediastinal fat close to the oesophagus.

Apical

This is a small gland that lies on the right side of the trachea just at the bifurcation of the accessory bronchus.

Afferents of the lung lymph nodes come from the heart, pericardium, lungs and pleura.

Intestines

Mesenteric
A large number of elongated nodes that lie in the mesentery along the lesser curvature of the intestines and about 5 cm from them. Afferents are from the small intestine. The chyle from the intestines flows through these nodes.

Gastrics
These are numerous but their sizes and numbers are variable. Afferents are from the walls of the stomach and spleen.

Liver

Portal (hepatic)
Embedded in fat at the hilum of the liver. Afferents are from the liver.

Lymph nodes of the bovine and sheep carcass (Figs 6.3–6.5)

Middle cervicals
Situated in the middle of the neck on each side of the trachea. They vary in number, from one to seven.

Presternal (one each side)
Situated superficially at the entrance of the thorax on the anterior border of the 1st ribs.

Suprasternals
Situated between the costal cartilages and covered by the transversus thoracis muscle. Afferent vessels are from the diaphragm, pleura, pericardium, peritoneum and chest muscles.

Prepectorals (one of each in each side)
Superficial and deep. Situated below the presternal nodes anterior to the middle of the 1st ribs. Afferent vessels are from middle cervicals, presternal, prescapular and axillary nodes and lymph vessels of head and neck.

Axillary (brachial) (one each side)
Situated between the scapula and the space between the 1st and 2nd ribs, about midway between the vertebral column and sternum. The afferent vessels come from the outer wall of the thorax and the scapula.

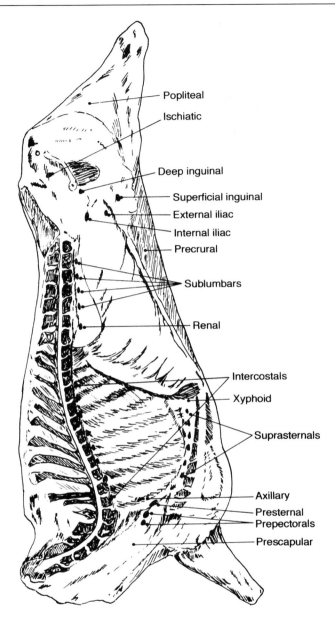

Fig. 6.3 Lymph nodes of ox carcass.

Prescapular (one each side)

Situated on the outside of the carcass embedded in fat, about a hand's breadth in front of the shoulder joints. The afferent vessels come from the cervical nodes, the shoulder, and upper foreleg.

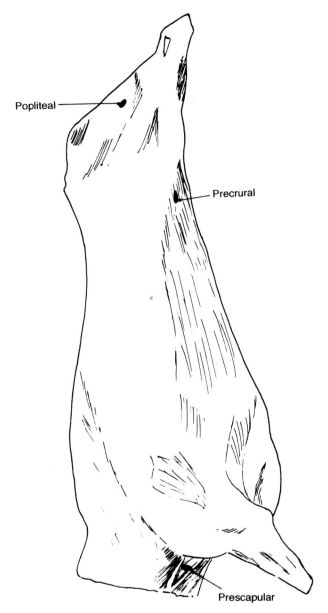

Fig. 6.4   Lymph nodes of ox carcass.

Intercostals or dorsals
Situated deep in the intercostal spaces at the junctions of the ribs with the vertebrae. Afferents are from muscles of dorsal region, intercostal muscles, ribs and
parietal pleurae.

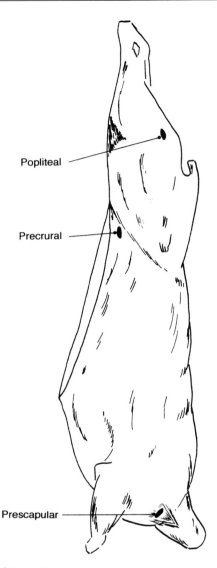

Fig. 6.5   Lymph nodes of sheep carcass.

Xyphoid (one each side)

Situated just inside the highest points of the sternum, in loose fat in the insides of the xyphoid cartilage. Afferents are from pleurae, diaphragm and ribs.

Subdorsals

Chains of small glands situated in the loose connective tissue between the aorta and the dorsal vertebrae. Afferents are from the dorsal vertebrae and the dorsal muscles.

Sublumbars
Chains of small nodes on the side of the posterior aorta close to the lumbar vertebrae. Afferents are from abdominal wall, lumbar muscles and organs in the pelvic cavity.

Renal (one each side)
Situated in kidney fat at hilum of kidney. Afferents are from kidney and adrenal gland.

Internal and external iliac (one of each in each side)
Situated in fat at entrance to the pelvis. Afferents are from muscles of the sub-lumbqra region, pelvis, thigh, urogenital tract and peritoneum.

Deep inguinal (one each side)
At the inlet of the pelvis in the femoral canals. Situated in fat about 5 cm under the pubic tubercle. Afferents are from the hind limb and the abdominal wall.

Ischiatic (one each side)
Lies on the outer aspects of the sacro-sciatic ligament. Exposed by deep incisions on vertical line midway between the posterior part of the ischium and the sacrum. Afferents are from the popliteal node and the sacro-coccygeal muscles.

Precrural (one each side)
Situated on the outside of the carcass and is embedded in fat. It is exposed by incisions made at the edge of the tensor fascia lata, about 18 cm down from the apex of the muscle. Afferent vessels are from the skin, prepuce and superficial muscles.

Superficial inguinal (one each side)
In the male is situated in the cod fat at the neck of the scrotum. afferent vessels are from the external genitals, the abdominal wall and the femoral region.

Supramammary (one each side)
In the female is situated above and behind the udder. Afferents are from the udder.

Popliteal (one each side)
Situated deep in the popliteal space, in the centre of the round of beef, immediately above and behind the stifle joint, embedded in fat. Afferents are from lower part of leg and foot.

Lymph nodes of the deer and goat

The positions of the lymph nodes are similar to those of the sheep.

Lymph nodes in pigs that differ from those in cattle (Fig. 6.6)

Submaxillaries are the main nodes in the head of the pig and lie under the sub-maxillary salivary glands.

Retropharyngeals are much smaller than in cattle and if head is removed may be left on carcass very close to the 1st cervical vertebra or atlas.

Cervicals form a more or less continuous chain running towards the prescapular.

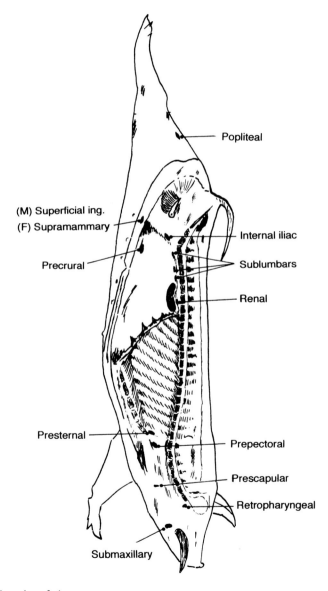

Fig. 6.6 Lymph nodes of pig carcass.

Prescapulars are cut from the inside of the carcass in pigs.

Axillaries, suprasternals and *intercostals* are very small or absent.

Precrurals are cut from inside in pigs through the abdominal muscles at the same level as the iliacs.

Popliteals are more superficial in pigs and lie in the midline, equidistant from the point of the hock and anus.

Supremammaries or *superficial inguinals* lie in the middle of the belly fat, level with the last teat.

Presternals are large and lie on the thoracic surface of the 1st ribs.

Gastrics. Three or four large glands on the lesser curvature of the stomach.

Mesenterics. Relatively farther away from the lesser curvature of the intestines and more lobulated.

Lymph nodes of the horse

The position of the lymph nodes is very similar to that of cattle. However, the nodes are small and occur in groups unlike the large individual nodes of cattle, e.g. the submaxillary lumph nodes are arranged in two elongated groups that join to give a V-formation.

Chapter 7
Respiratory System

This is the system by which the body tissues take up oxygen and dispose of carbon dioxide. Inspired air is taken into the lungs whee it immediately comes almost into contact with the blood, being separated only by a thin membrane. The blood takes in O_2 from the air and passes CO_2 back into the air. This air is then expired and fresh air taken in again with the next inspiration.

Inspiration

This is a muscular act. The inspiratory muscles increase the size of the chest cavity and form a vacuum between the lungs and the chest walls. Atmospheric pressure forces air into the lungs. The muscles used in inspiration are (1) the diaphragm, which is the large muscular sheet that separates the chest from the abdomen; (2) the intercostal muscles, which are the muscles between the ribs; and (3) the abdominal muscles. When the chest cavity is enlarged, the lungs fill with air and fill this cavity.

Expiration

This is the reverse action. The muscles relax, the chest cavity reduces in size and the lungs contract partly by their own elasticity and partly by reduction of the chest cavity. The air is thus forced out of the lungs.

The external respirtory apparatus comprises the nostrils, the nasal cavity, the pharynx, the larynx, the trachea, the bronchi and the lungs.

The nasal cavity opens externally at the nostrils and communicates behind with the pharynx and larynx. It contains the turbinate bones and is divided symmetrically by the nasal septum.

The pharynx is a common passage for air and food.

The larynx (Figs 7.1 and 7.2)

This is a short tube that connects the pharynx with the trachea. It is a complex valvular apparatus, which regulates the volume of air passing through the tract,

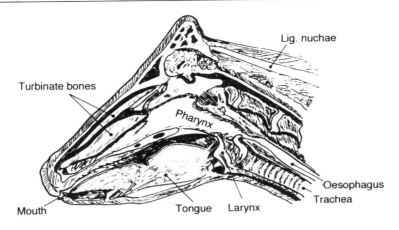

Fig. 7.1 Section of an ox head.

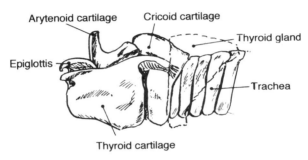

Fig. 7.2 Larynx of ox.

prevents aspiration of foreign material and, as it contains the vocal cords, is the chief organ of voice.

It is composed of three single cartilages and one pair:

(1) The cricoid cartilage – shaped like a signet ring
(2) The thyroid cartilage – composed of a body and two wings
(3) The epiglottic cartilage or epiglottis is situated above the body of the thyroid cartilage and curves towards the root of the tongue.
(4) The arytenoid cartilages are situated on either side, in front of the cricoid.

In normal dressing of the carcass the larynx is left on the head in cattle, sheep and horses, but is left attached to the trachea in pigs.

The trachea and the lungs

The trachea

The trachea extends from the larynx to the roots of the lungs where it divides into right, left and apical bronchi. It is kept permanently open by a series of incomplete cartilaginous rings embedded in its wall. There is no apical bronchus in the horse.

The lungs

The lungs, right and left, occupy most of the thoracic cavity. The right lung in all animals is larger than the left. The lungs are divided into a varying number of lobes. The lung tissue crepitates when pressed between the finger and thumb and floats in water. In contrast, fetal lung tissue is: (1) firmer and does not crepitate, (2) sinks in water, and (3) is purple in colour as opposed to pink.

When the thoracic cavity is opened, the lungs collapse to about one-third of their original size.

Ox trachea and lungs *(Fig. 7.3)*

(1) Trachea – has dorsal ridge, about 50 rings and averages about 65 cm in length. Calibre 3.5–5 cm
(2) Left lung has three lobes, right has four or five
(3) Right accessory bronchus, going to the apical lobe
(4) Lung lobulation well marked
(5) Weight 2.5–3 kg.

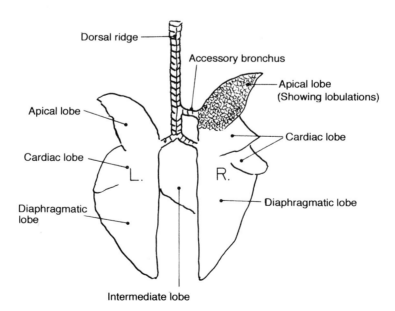

Fig. 7.3 Lungs of ox.

Sheep trachea and lungs

(1) Trachea similar to ox but, of course, much smaller. Average length 22–25 cm. Calibre 1.5 cm
(2) Consistency more dense and leathery to the touch
(3) Lung lobulation indistinct
(4) Weight 350 g–1 kg.

Goat trachea and lungs *(similar to sheep)*

Pig trachea, lungs and larynx *(Fig. 7.4)*

(1) Trachea about 15–20 cm long, 32–35 rings, which overlap dorsally and therefore no tracheal ridge
(2) Left three lobes, right three or four
(3) Right accessory bronchus
(4) Lung very compressible
(5) Lobulation distinct
(6) Interarytenoid cartilage present in larynx
(7) Weight 350–450 g.

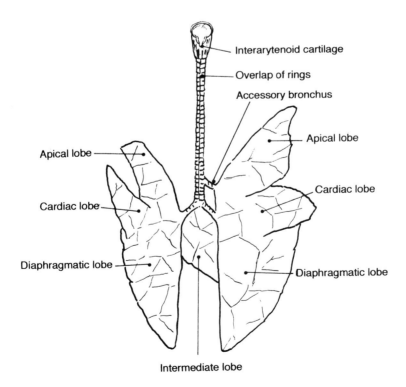

Fig. 7.4 Lungs of pig.

Horse trachea and lungs *(Fig. 7.5)*

(1) Trachea longer than ox – average 75–80 cm and calibre 5 cm, 50–60 rings and no tracheal ridge
(2) Left two lobes, right three lobes, butlobes indistinct and not divided by deep fissures
(3) No accessory bronchus
(4) No surface lobulation
(5) Much longer than ox
(6) Weight variable.

NB Because of the large variations in sizes, e.g. between a heavy draught horse and a small pony, the weight of lungs has not been included.

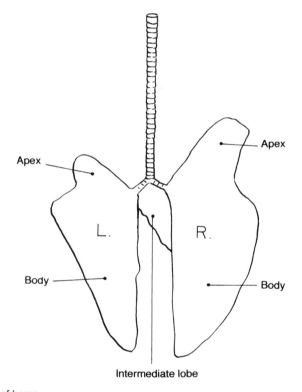

Fig. 7.5 Lungs of horse.

Deer lungs, larynx and trachea *(Fig. 7.6)*

(1) Trachea is much longer relatively than sheep; 60 rings on average, and no obvious tracheal ridge
(2) Consistency not so dense as sheep
(3) Lobulation indistinct.

NB Size and weight not included because of species variation.

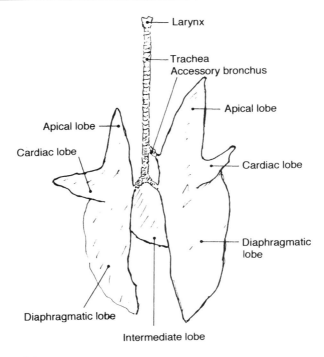

Larynx

Trachea
Accessory bronchus

Apical lobe

Apical lobe

Cardiac lobe

Cardiac lobe

Diaphragmatic
lobe

Diaphragmatic lobe

Intermediate lobe

Fig. 7.6 Lungs of deer.

The pleura

The *pleura* is a continuous, thin, double, serous membrane that is firmly attached to the walls of the thorax and its contents, except for the heart, which has its own serous covering – the pericardium (p. 25). The free surface is very smooth and glistening in appearance. It is lubricated by the *pleural fluid* so that opposing surfaces glide over each other. It is well supplied with blood and lymph vessels. For the sake of convenience it is divided into various parts:

(1) The *visceral pleura* covers the lungs, except at the hilums where the bronchi, blood vessels and nerves enter the lungs.
(2) The *parietal pleura* covers the walls of the thorax. The part attached to the thoracic surface of the diaphragm is called the *diaphragmatic pleura*.
(3) The *mediastinal pleura* covers the blood vessels, the oesophagus, the lymph nodes, etc. in the mediastinal space. The part that is attached to the pericardium is the *pericardiac pleura*.

Chapter 8
Digestive System

Digestion comprises the operations to which food is subjected from the time it is eaten until it is absorbed. The materials required for the life of the body are supplied by the circulating fluids, blood and lympth. This requires that the nutrients be soluble in water or be so finely divided that they can be transported in a liquid medium. Since the food as it is taken into the body is not in this condition, considerable changes must take place before it can be transported in the blood. These changes as a whole constitute digestion. The food, in addition to undergoing mechanical and chemical digestion, must also be transported along the alimentary tract and the products of digestion must be transferred through membranes from the lumen of the intestine into the capillaries of the portal circulation and lymphatics.

The organs of digestion, known collectively as the digestive or alimentary tract, are the mouth, oesophagus, stomach, small and large intestines and various accessory structures associated with those organs.

Chemical aspects of digestion

Digestive secretions

(1) *Saliva* is the first secretion encountered by food in its progress through the alimentary tract. It is secreted mainly by three pairs of glands – the salivary glands:

(a) submaxillary glands
(b) parotid salivary glands
(c) sublingual salivary glands

The salivary glands empty their secretions through ducts that lead into various parts of the mouth. Saliva contains the starch-splitting amylase enzyme *ptyalin*.

(2) *Gastric juice* – a complex fluid secreted by various types of glands situated in different parts of the lining or mucuous membrane of the stomach. Gastric juice contains *hydrochloric acid* and the enzymes *pepsin*, *rennin* and *lipase*.

(3) *Pancreatic juice* is produced by the pancreas from which it enters the intestine by means of two ducts. It contains three main enzymes, *lipase*, *trypsinogen* and *amylase*.
(4) *Intestinal juice* is secreted by the cells of the mucous membrane of the small intestine. It contains the enzymes, *aminotripeptidase, dipeptidase, maltase, lactase* and *invertase*.
(5) *Bile* is produced by the liver and enters the intestine by the bile duct from the liver. It contains two bile salts, *bilirubin* and *biliverdin*. They play an important part in the digestion and absorption of fat. They are also converted by bacteria into *stercobilin*, a pigment that colours the faeces.

Bacteria in the alimentary tract also play an important part in the digestion of food, especially in the digestive system of ruminants, e.g. cattle and sheep.

The alimentary canal

This is a tube that extends from the lips to the anus. It has a complete lining of mucuous membrane, external to which is an almost continuous muscular coat. The abdominal portion of the tube is largely covered with a serous membrane – the visceral peritoneum. The canal consists of the following consecutive parts: (1) the mouth, (2) the pharynx, (3) the oesophagus, (4) the stomach, (5) the small intestine, (6) the large intestine, and (7) the anus.

The mouth

The mouth is the first part of the alimentary canal. It contains the tongue and teeth and opens behind into the pharynx, or back of the throat, which in turn opens into both the trachea or windpipe and the oesophagus or gullet. The roof of the mouth consists of the hard palate in front, which in the ox and sheep is more or less pigmented and ridged, and the soft palate behind. Also in the ox and sheep the inside of cheeks and parts of the lips have a large number of conical papillae. The ox, sheep, deer and goat have no upper incisor teeth but have a *dental pad*. This is the most anterior part of the hard palate. It consists of a thick layer of dense connective tissue that has a thick horny epithelial covering. The soft palate is long in the horse, so long in fact that the horse is unable to breathe through the mouth.

The pharynx

The pharynx is a musculo-membraneous sac that is common to the digestive and respiratory tracts and lies at the back of the mouth.

The tongue

Ox tongue (Fig. 8.1)

(1) Rough tip – horny filiform (conical) papillae
(2) Pronounced dorsal prominence on dorsum
(3) 10–14 vallate papillae on either side of mid-line of prominent dorsum form a long narrow group
(4) Sometimes spotted with black pigment.

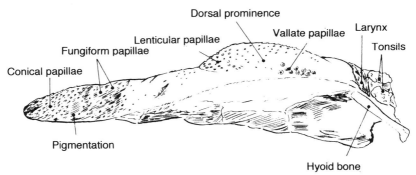

Fig. 8.1 Tongue of ox (× 0.25).

Sheep and goat tongue (Fig. 8.2)

(1) Tip notched – filiform papillae not horny
(2) Pigmentation common.

Differentiated from calf tongue by being narrower, dorsal prominence more marked, surface smoother and tip rounded.

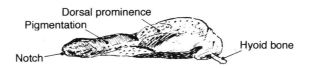

Fig. 8.2 Tongue of sheep (× 0.5).

Pig tongue (Fig. 8.3)

(1) Long and narrow and no dorsal ridge
(2) One or two marked vallate papillae each side of mid-line near base
(3) Fungiform papillae on sides of tongue are very prominent
(4) Soft, long, pointed papillae directed backwards on root
(5) Evidence of scalding on tip, i.e. the mucous membrane is torn and ragged.

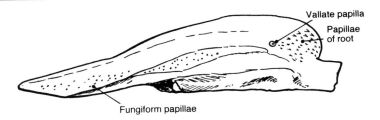

Fig. 8.3   Tongue of pig (× 0.5).

Horse tongue (Fig. 8.4)

(1)   Long, flat and smooth with spatulate end
(2)   One vallate papilla each side
(3)   Never pigmented.

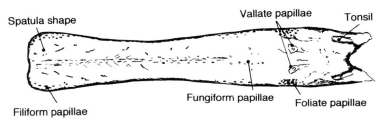

Fig. 8.4   Tongue of horse (× 0.2).

Deer tongue (Fig. 8.5)

(1)   Tip smooth and slightly notched
(2)   Tongue slightly broader at anterior end but not spatulate like horse tongue
(3)   Pronounced dorsal prominence
(4)   Fungiform papillae are numerous just in front of and at sides of dorsum
(5)   Numerous flattened papillae on top of dorsum
(6)   Not pigmented.

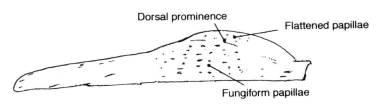

Fig. 8.5   Tongue of deer (× 0.5).

The oesophagus

the oesophagus is the muscular tube that leads from the mouth to the stomach
(see Fig. 7.1).

The tonsils

The tonsils are composed of lymphoid tissue.

Ox tonsils lie in the tonsillar sinuses in the anterior pillars of the soft palate lateral to the root of the tongue. they are bean-shaped and about 3–4 cm in length.

Sheep tonsils (Fig. 8.6) are bean-shaped, about 12 mm in length and are similar in position to the ox tonsils.

Goat tonsils are similar to those of the sheep.

Pig tonsils are not compact in shape but are represented by tonsillar tissue in the soft palate and root of the tongue.

Horse tonsils, as in the pig, are not compact tonsils. They are represented by a series of masses of lymphoid tissue that extend backward about 10 cm on each side of the root of the tongue.

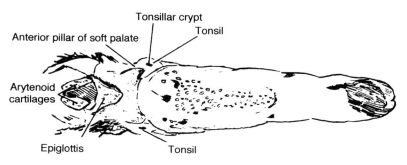

Fig. 8.6   Sheep tongue showing position of tonsils.

The stomach

Ox stomach

In cattle the stomach (Figs 8.7 and 8.8) consists of four compartments: rumen or 1st stomach; reticulum (honeycomb) or 2nd stomach; omasum (manyplies) or 3rd stomach; abomasum or 4th stomach. This is the true stomach and secretes gastric juice. The other three stomachs are really just dilatations of the oesophagus and produce no gastric juice.

In adult cattle the rumen occupies three-quarters of the abdominal cavity.

A feature of the calf stomach is the relatively large size of the abomasum as compared with the small size of the rumen, which only enlarges when the calf is weaned and begins to eat solid food, grass, hay, etc. Rennet is obtained commercially from the calf abomasum or vell. Calf vells are sold commercially as dried, blown or flat vells.

Sheep, goat and deer stomach

All these animals are also ruminants and therefore the stomachs will be similar to

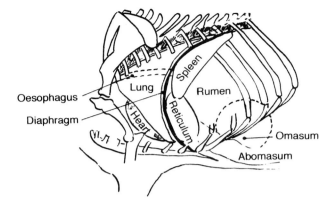

Fig. 8.7   Thoracic and abdominal viscera of ox.

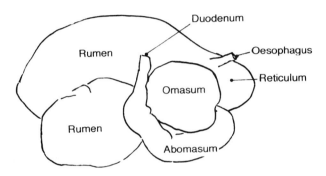

Fig. 8.8   Stomach of ox.

that of the ox. The stomachs will vary in size due to the relative size differences between the different animals.

Pig stomach

The pig stomach (Fig. 8.9) is simple, and semilunar in shape with a small pocket or diverticulum at the cardiac end. The mucuous membrane at the cardiac end is

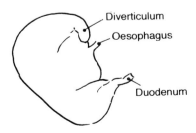

Fig. 8.9   Stomach of pig.

pale grey, the central area reddish brown, becoming paler and corrugated towards the pylorus. Hodges are prepared from pigs' stomachs.

Horse stomach

The horse stomach (Fig. 8.10) is simple and consists of a sharply curved, U-shaped sac, the right part being, however, much shorter than the left one. It is relatively small.

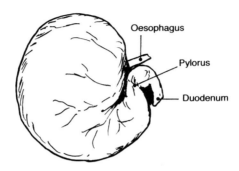

Fig. 8.10   Stomach of horse.

The intestines

The *small intestine* starts at the outlet of the stomach – the *pylorus* – and terminates at the entrance of the caecum at the *ileo-caecal valve*.

It is clearly divided into two parts, a fixed and a mesenteric part. The fixed part is called the *duodenum* and the mesenteric part is conventionally divided into the *jejunum* and *ileum*.

The *large intestine* extends from the end of the *ileum* to the *anus*. It differs from the small intestine in its greater size and in having a more fixed position. In the horse it is sacculated for the most part, possessing longitudinal bands. In the ox there are no longitudinal bands, and it is not sacculated and is much smaller in calibre.

It is divided into the *caecum*, which has a blind end, the *colon* and *rectum*.

Average lengths of the various intestines are given in Table 8.1.

Table 8.1   Average lengths of intestines.

	Small intestines (m)	Large intestines (m)
Cattle	36	9
Horse	24	6
Sheep	25	6
Pig	17	5
Deer	25	6

The ratio of the length of small intestines to large intestines is about 4:1.

Accessory organs

The liver

The functions of the liver are as follows:

(1)   The liver stores excess carbohydrates as *glycogen* and regulates the amount of glucose in the blood.
(2)   The liver prepares fat for utilisation as a source of energy.
(3)   The liver deaminates *amino acids* not needed for building up new proto-plasm. From some amino acids it is able to manufacture *fibrinogen* and probably *albumin proteins* of blood.
(4)   During the 'wear and tear' of the body a certain amount of protoplasm is broken down and forms *nitrogenous waste*. This passes in the blood to the liver where it is converted into *urea, creatinine* or *uric acid*. This waste then passes in the blood to the kidneys, where it is excreted.
(5)   The liver produces and secretes *bile*.
(6)   The liver stores vitamin B_{12} – an anti-anaemic principle. The liver discharges this into the blood in which it passes to the bone marrow where it has some effect on the formation of new red corpuscles.
(7)   The liver stores iron.
(8)   The liver is a large organ and does a great deal of work. Consequently it produces much energy in the form of heat, which is important in maintaining body temperature.

With the exception of the horse liver, which is purplish, the livers of all food animals are reddish-brown.

Ox liver (Fig. 8.11)

(1)   Three lobes; the thin, left lobe is indistinctly divided from the thicker, right and a caudate lobe. In young animals the liver is almost circular in outline. As the animal ages the liver elongates and becomes more oval in shape with a narrowing between the right and left lobe.
(2)   The gall bladder is pear-shaped. If it is removed during dressing, the area of removal is obvious as the peritoneal covering is torn or part of the liver has been cut off.
(3)   Weight 6–7 kg.

Sheep liver (Fig. 8.12)

(1)   Similar to ox but caudate lobe is more pointed and all edges are sharp
(2)   Deeper division between lobes
(3)   Gall bladder is cigar-shaped
(4)   Weight 500–700 g.

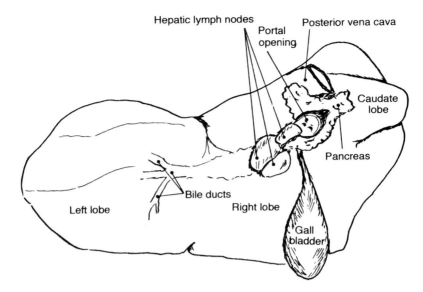

Fig. 8.11   Liver of cow (× 0.2).

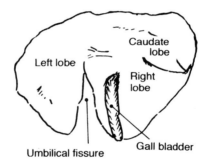

Fig. 8.12   Liver of sheep (× 0.2).

Calf liver (Fig. 8.13)
The calf liver has rounder edges and the caudate lobe has blunt end extending beyond edge of liver. The remains of the umbilical vein are still present.

Goat liver
The liver of goat is similar to that of sheep.

Pig liver (Fig. 8.14)

(1)   Five lobes
(2)   Large lobules giving morocco leather appearance
(3)   Gall bladder is pear-shaped
(4)   Weight 1 kg (porker); 3.5 kg (sow).

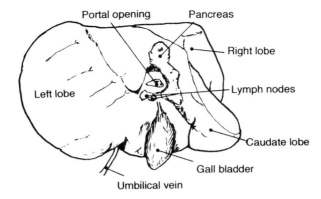

Fig. 8.13   Liver of calf (× 0.2).

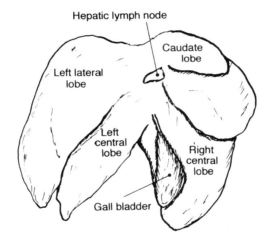

Fig. 8.14   Liver of pig (× 0.2).

Horse liver (Fig. 8.15)

(1)   Three indistinct lobes
(2)   Caudate is triangular
(3)   No gall bladder
(4)   Purplish in colour
(5)   Middle lobe has three small fissures on its free edge, producing the so called 'fingers'
(6)   Weight variable.

Red deer liver (Fig. 8.16)

(1)   Three lobes
(2)   No gall bladder

(3) Umbilical fissure small
(4) Portal opening small

NB There is a big variation in the shapes and sizes of the livers of the various species. The outstanding feature of all deer livers is the absence of a gall bladder.

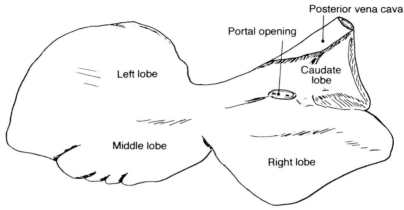

Fig. 8.15 Liver of horse (× 0.12).

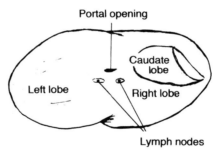

Fig. 8.16 Liver of red deer (× 0.5).

The pancreas

The pancreas (gut-sweetbread) in the ox is attached to the posterior surface of the liver. It is yellowish brown, lobulated and the shape of an oak leaf. In the pig it is paler in colour and is found between loops of the small intestine in the region of the kidneys, and often a portion of pancreas can be found in the pig carcass attached to the kidney region. The pancreas produces pancreatic juice, conveyed to the small intestine by the pancreatic duct, and it also produces insulin, which is absorbed directly into the bloodstream. The pancreas is thus both an ordinary gland with a duct and a ductless gland.

The spleen (or melt)

This is considered here, although it is not part of the digestive system, because it is contained in the abdomen.

The spleen is an integral part of the lymphatic and blood vascular systems. It is a specially designed lymphatic tissue interposed in the bloodstream and is an important organ for:

(1) Removing foreign material from the bloodstream, including disease-producing organisms and worn-out blood cells
(2) Producing lymphocytes and other blood cells
(3) Producing antibodies
(4) Storing iron (from red blood corpuscles)
(5) Storing blood and maintaining a constant circulating blood volume.

Ox spleen (Fig. 8.17)

(1) Elongated oval shape
(2) Bluish in colour
(3) Rounded edges in young animals
(4) White lymph follicles (malpighian corpuscles) that are easily seen on cross-section
(5) Weight 1 kg.

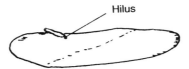

Fig. 8.17   Spleen of ox (× 0.1).

Sheep and goat spleen (Fig. 8.18)

(1) Oyster-shaped
(2) Reddish brown in colour
(3) Soft and elastic to touch
(4) Weight 50–90 g.

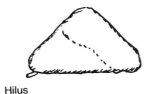

Fig. 8.18   Spleen of sheep (× 0.3).

Pig spleen (Fig. 8.19)

(1) Elongated tongue shape
(2) Three edges and reddish in colour
(3) Triangular in cross-section
(4) Longitudinal ridge with fat-filled omentum attached
(5) Weight 200 g.

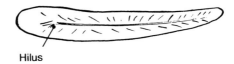

Hilus

Fig. 8.19   Spleen of pig (× 0.2).

Horse spleen (Fig. 8.20)

(1) Flat and sickle-shaped
(2) Bluish in colour
(3) Weight variable.

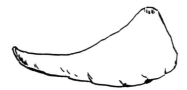

Fig. 8.20   Spleen of horse (× 0.1).

Deer spleen (Fig. 8.21)

(1) Flat and oval shaped, length to width ratio of 3:2
(2) Reddish brown in colour
(3) Soft and elastic to touch
(4) Weight variable.

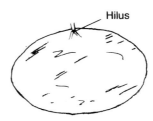

Hilus

Fig. 8.21   Spleen of deer (× 0.5).

The peritoneum

The peritoneum is the thin, double, serous membrane that lines the abdominal cavity and part of the pelvic cavity, and covers to a greater or lesser extent the contained viscera. In the male it is a completely closed sac, but in the female there are two small openings in it. These are the abdominal orifices of the fallopian tubes, which communicate with the uterus and so indirectly with the exterior.

The peritoneal cavity is only a potential one, since the opposing walls are only separated by the serous fluid (secreted by the membrane), which acts as a lubricant. It is essential not to confuse the peritoneal cavity with the abdominal cavity. The organs are all extraperitoneal.

The free surface of the peritoneum has a glistening appearance and is very smooth. It is moistened by peritoneal fluid and thus friction is reduced to a minimum during the movements iof the viscera. The peritoneum that lines the walls of the abdomen and part of the pelvis is called the *parietal layer* and that covering the viscera the *visceral layer*. The connecting folds are termed omenta, mesenteries and ligaments.

An *omentum* is a fold of peritoneum that passes from the stomach to other viscera.

A *mesentery* is a fold of peritoneum that attaches the intestines to the dorsal wall of the abdomen.

A *ligament* is a fold of peritoneum that passes between viscera, other than parts of the digestive tube, or which connects them with the abdominal wall. (not to be confused with ligaments attached to bones.)

The *pelvic peritoneum* is continuous in front with that of the abdomen. It lines the pelvic cavity for a variable distance backwards and is then reflected on to the viscera and from one organ to another.

Chapter 9
Urogenital System

The urogenital system consists of (1) the urinary organs, and (2) the genital organs.

The urinary organs

The urinary organs, which produce and remove *urine*, are the *kidneys*, *ureters*, *bladder* and *urethra*. The kidneys produce the urine, which is conveyed to the bladder by the ureters. The urethra conveys the urine from the bladder to the penis in the male and to the vagina in the female.

The kidneys

The typical kidney is bean-shaped and covered by a thin, tough, fibrous capsule that continues inwardly at an indentation on the medial surface, the *hilum*. The renal artery enters and the renal vein and *ureter* exit at the hilum. The ureter is expanded within the kidney as the *renal pelvis*, which in turn divides into smaller conduits, the *renal calyxes*. Each calyx fits around the apex of a pyramidal structure, the *renal pyramid*. Each pyramid is the site of the junction of many smaller kidney ducts that converge upon its apex, the *papilla*. The papillae deliver urine into the calyxes and pelvis.

Ox kidneys (Fig. 9.1)

(1)   Lobulated, 15–25 lobules
(2)   Left kidney is three-sided, and movable in the abdomen; right kidney is elliptical and fixed in the abdomen

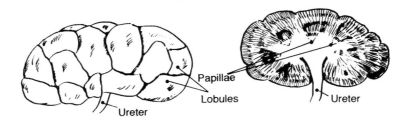

Fig. 9.1   Kidney of ox (whole and bisected, × 0.2).

(3) Reddish brown in colour
(4) 15–25 renal papillae
(5) No renal pelvis
(6) Weight 280–340 g.

Sheep and goat kidneys (Fig. 9.2)

(1) Bean-shaped
(2) Dark brown in colour
(3) One renal papilla and pelvis present
(4) Weight 57–85 g.

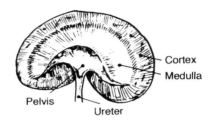

Fig. 9.2 Kidney of sheep (bisected, × 0.3).

Pig kidneys (Fig. 9.3)

(1) Elongated, bean-shaped
(2) Thinner and flatter than others
(3) Reddish brown in colour
(4) 10–12 renal papillae and renal pelvis is present
(5) Weight 85–170 g

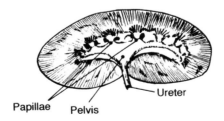

Fig. 9.3 Kidney of pig (bisected, × 0.3).

Horse kidneys (Fig. 9.4)

(1) Right kidney is heart-shaped
(2) Left kidney is bean-shaped
(3) One renal papilla
(4) Weight variable.

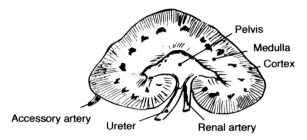

Fig. 9.4   Right kidney of horse (bisected × 0.3).

Deer kidneys (Fig. 9.5)

(1)   Bean-shaped, slightly more elongated than sheep
(2)   Dark brown in colour
(3)   6 renal papillae and pelvis present.

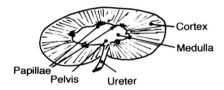

Fig. 9.5   Kidney of deer (× 0.5).

The genital organs

The genital organs form, develop, and expel the products of the reproductive glands.

The male genital organs

These comprise the following (Fig. 9.6):

(1)   Two *testicles* – the essential reproductive organs in which sperm are produced.
(2)   The *ductus deferens* – the ducts of the testicles
(3)   The *vesiculae seminales* or seminal vesicles
(4)   The *prostate* – a musculo-glandular organ
(5)   Two *bulbo-urethral glands*
(6)   The *urethra*, a canal that transmits the generative and urinary secretions
(7)   The *penis*.

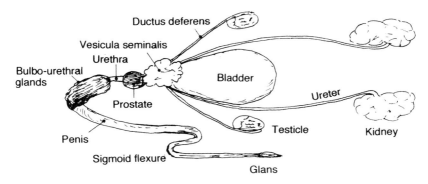

Fig. 9.6 Urogenital system of bull.

Bull testicles (Fig. 9.7)

(1) Elongated, oval in outline, weight 280–340 g
(2) Parenchyma yellowish in colour
(3) Heavy veining
(4) Epididymis is narrow and is closely attached along the posterior border. The head is long and curved over the upper extremity and one-third the way down the anterior border.

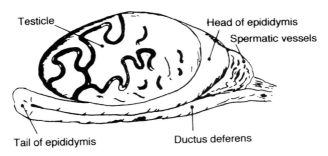

Fig. 9.7 Testicle of bull (× 0.3).

Ram testicles (Fig. 9.8)

(1) Similar to bull but are relatively larger, pear-shaped and more rounded, weight 250–280 g
(2) Light veining.

Billy-goat testicles (as ram)

Boar testicles (Fig. 9.9)

(1) Very large and irregularly elliptical
(2) Parenchyma is greyish, or brown

(3) Branched main vein
(4) Interlobular tissue is abundant and lobulations are distinct
(5) Epididymis is well developed and forms a blunt conical projection at both ends of the testicle.

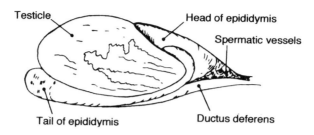

Fig. 9.8 Testicle of ram (× 0.5).

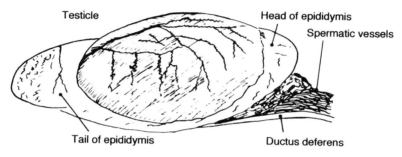

Fig. 9.9 Testicle of boar (× 0.3).

Horse testicles (Fig. 9.10)

(1) Relatively smaller than those of the other animals, measuring 10 cm × 6.4 cm, weight about 220 g (variable)
(2) Parenchyma is reddish grey
(3) Ovoid in shape but are compressed from side to side
(4) Light veining

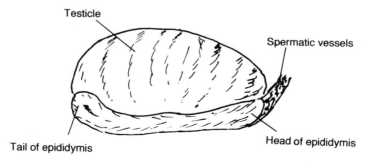

Fig. 9.10 Testicle of stallion (× 0.6).

(5)   The body of the epididymis is loosely attached but the head and tail are more firmly attached to the lower thirds of the upper and lower extremities.

Deer testicles (Fig. 9.11)

(1)   Elongated oval in outline
(2)   Parenchyma is yellowish in colour
(3)   Very light veining
(4)   Epididymis is very narrow and loosely attached along posterior border, but head and tail are firmly attached.

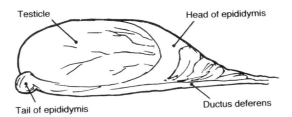

Testicle   Head of epididymis

Tail of epididymis   Ductus deferens

Fig. 9.11   Testicle of deer (× 0.5).

The female genital organs

These comprise the following:

(1)   The *two ovaries*, the essential reproductive glands, in which the eggs or ova are produced
(2)   The *uterine* or *fallopian tubes* which convey the ova to the uterus
(3)   The *uterus* in which the ovum develops
(4)   The *vagina*, a dilatable passage through which the fetus is expelled from the uterus
(5)   The *vulva*, the terminal segment of the genital tract, which serves also for the expulsion of urine
(6)   The *mammary glands*, which are in reality glands of the skin, but are so closely associated functionally with the generative organs proper that they are usually described with them

Uteri

The uterus, in which the ovum develops, is a Y-shaped muscular organ. It consists of a body, two horns or cornua and a neck. It is connected anteriorly with the fallopian tubes and posteriorly with the vagina.

Cow uterus (Fig. 9.12)

(1) This varies tremendously in size depending on whether pregnant or not and the duration of pregnasncy. As pregnancy progresses the uterus increases in size but the wall of the uterus gets progressively thinner due to the stretching.

(2) In the non-pregnant cow the uterus consists of a small body about 3–4 cm long and two horns or cornua about 35–40 cm long.

(3) When the horns are pulled apart there is a double fold of tissue at the base between them.

(4) On the mucous membrane there are approximately 100 oval prominences called cotyledons. These increase in size during pregnancy from about 15 mm to 10–12 cm in length. They also become pedunculated, pitted on the surface and have a spongy appearance.

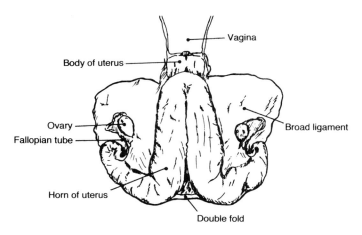

Fig. 9.12   Uterus of cow (non-pregnant, × 0.2).

Heifer uterus

(1) This is much smaller than the cow uterus and can be held in the palm of the hand.

(2) The cotyledons are small, oval, non-pedunculated, 15 × 18 mm and non-pitted.

Ewe uterus

(1) This is similar to the cow uterus but of course is very much smaller and the horns are relatively longer.

(2) When the horns are pulled apart there is a single fold of tissue and not double as in a cow.

(3) The cotyledons are much smaller, circular, pigmented and in pregnancy the centres are cupped.
(4) When pregnant the cotyledons can be seen through the wall of the uterus. This is not so in cattle.
(5) The horns are about 10 cm long and taper gradually towards the junctions with the fallopian tubes so that no clear distinction exists between them as it does in the cow.

Nanny-goat uterus (as ewe)

Sow uterus (Fig. 9.13)

(1) The body is about 5 cm long.
(2) The horns are extremely long, 1.2 m and flexous. If not pregnant they are coiled and appear very like the small intestine.
(3) There are no cotyledons.

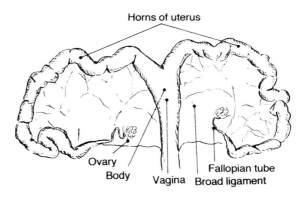

Fig. 9.13   Uterus of sow (non-pregnant, × 0.1).

Mare uterus (Fig. 9.14)

(1) The body of the uterus is 18–20 cm long and is flattened, so that in cross-section it is elliptical
(2) The horns are about 25 cm long in the non-pregnant mare and have blunt points.
(3) There are no cotyledons.

Deer uterus (Fig. 9.15)

(1) The body is relatively much longer than that of the cow or ewe.
(2) When the horns are pulled apart there is a single fold of tissue.
(3) There are nine cotyledons (four in each horn and one almost central where the body joins the horns.).

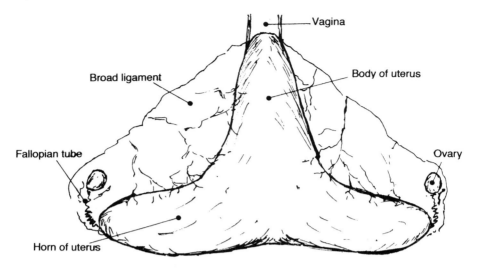

Fig. 9.14   Uterus of mare (non-pregnant, × 0.2).

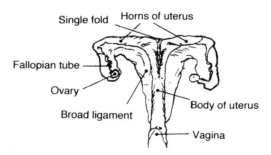

Fig. 9.15   Uterus of deer.

(4)   In the gravid uterus the cotyledons are large, oval to circular in outline, slightly flattened and with spitted sponge-like surfaces with no pigmentation.

NB Size not given owing to species variation.

Chapter 10
Nervous System

The nervous system may be divided into:

(1) The central nervous system – consisting of (1) the spinal cord, and (2) the brain.
(2) The peripheral nervous system – consisting of the cranial, spinal and peripheral nerves with their motor and sensory endings.

Spinal cord

The spinal cord is a hollow tube that runs in the spinal canal of the vertebral column and is therefore protected by bone. At the cranial end it expands to form the brain, which is protected by the skull. The spinal cord and the brain together form the central nervous system.

Between the bone and this central nervous system are three membranes called meninges:

(1) The *pia mater* – adherent to the brain and spinal cord. It carries small blood vessels to and from the central nervous system.
(2) The *arachnoid* – this is connected to the pia mater by delicate strands. The region between the two layers is the *subarachnoid space*, which is filled with the *cerebrospinal fluid*. This is formed mainly by the brain and it cushions the cord.
(3) The *dura mater* – this is a tough covering lining the inside of the skull and the neural canal.

The main function of the spinal cord is to convey messages to and from the brain to the muscles of the body.

The brain

The spinal cord swells out to form the brain composed of (Fig. 10.1):

(1) The *medulla oblongata* – this contains the centres for reflexes that control respiratory movements, the rate of the heart, swallowing, etc. on the posterior side of the medulla.

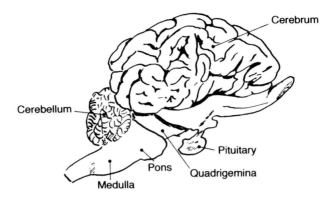

Fig. 10.1   Brain of ox.

(2)   the *cerebellum* has a ridged surface and is divided into two parts called the right and left hemispheres, which are joined by a bridge of nerve fibres called the *pons*. The cerebellum is the centre for reflexes that bring about muscular co-ordination.

The medulla oblongata and the cerebellum combine to form the hind-brain. Anterior to the cerebellum the brain stem swells out to form the four little swellings of the mid-brain.

(3)   The *quadrigemina* (or mid-brain) is the centre for reflexes connected with the eyes.

The brain stem then divides into:

(4)   The *cerebrum* (or fore-brain). This is composed of two large cerebral hemispheres. The cerebrum contains the higher centres for consciousness, reasoning, memory, voluntary movements, sight, hearing, etc.

The eye

The eye (Fig. 10.2) comprises the eyeball, the optic nerve and certain accessory organs, i.e. muscles, eyelids, conjunctiva and the lacrimal apparatus. The lacrimal apparatus comprises:

(1)   The lacrimal gland, which secretes the clear lacrimal fluid (tears)
(2)   the excretory ducts of the gland
(3)   the two lacrimal ducts, lacrimal sac and naso-lacrimal duct, which receive the fluid and convey it to the nostril.

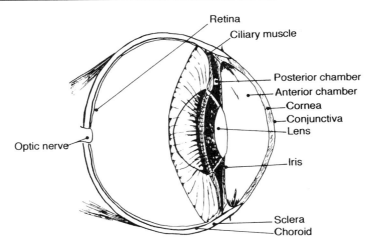

Fig. 10.2 Eye of horse.

The eyeball is protected in front by the eyelids and conjunctiva. The anterior transparent part is formed by the cornea and the posterior opaque part by the sclera. This is a dense fibrous membrane, which forms about four-fifths of the fibrous tunic. It is generally white but may have a bluish tinge in its thinner parts. Its inner surface is attached to the choroid. Inside the choroid is the retina, the light-sensitive part of the eye, on which the lens focuses objects seen. The retina then transmits this information to the brain via the optic nerve.

The *iris* is a muscular diaphragm placed in front of the lens and is visible through the cornea. The iris is the coloured part of the eye.

The *lens* is a biconvex, transparent body that divides the eye into anterior and posterior parts. The lens focuses objects seen on the retina and is acted upon by the ciliary muscle.

The *anterior chamber* is enclosed in front by the cornea and behind by the iris and lens. It is filled by the aqueous humour, which is a clear fluid.

The *posterior chamber* is a small annular space, triangular in cross-section, which is bounded in front by the iris, behind by the peripheral part of the lens and its ligaments and externally by the ciliary processes. It is filled by vitreous humour.

The ear

The ear (Fig. 10.3), or organ of hearing, consists of three natural divisions: (1) external, (2) middle, and (3) internal.

External ear

The external ear consists of (1) an auricle, a funnel-like organ that collects the sound waves, and (2) the external auditory meatus that conveys these waves to

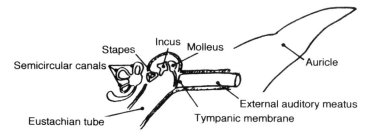

Fig. 10.3   Ear.

the tympanic membrane or drum that separates the external ear from the middle ear.

Middle ear

The middle ear consists of the tympanic cavity, auditory ossicles and the Eustachian tube, which extends to the pharynx. The auditory ossicles consist of a chain of three very small bones, malleus, incus and stapes, which convey the vibrations of the ear drum to the internal ear.

Internal ear

The internal ear consists of (1) a complex membranous sac lined with auditory cells that convey information (sounds) to the auditory nerve and so to the brain, (2) the semicircular canals, which are the organs of balance.

Chapter 11
Endocrine System

The *endocrine* or *ductless glands* synthesise *hormones*, which are secreted directly into the blood as it passes through the glands. The hormones are complex chemicals that have highly specific functions. Their concentration in the blood is always minute but the effects can be profound. Their actions are to control body growth, develop sex characteristics and stabilise the body functions. They are broken down in the liver and excreted in the urine.

Ductless glands

Pituitary gland

The pituitary gland is situated on the lower aspect of the cerebrum to which it is attached by a short stalk. In the bovine it is oval in outline, flattened and measures 2 cm in width. It rests in a small pit of bone formed by the base of the skull. Because its hormones partly control the other endocrine glands, it is sometimes called the 'master gland'. The anterior part produces at least six active principles and the posterior part two.

The anterior hormones are:

(1) *Somatotrophin* – stimulates growth
(2) *Thyrotrophin* – stimulates the thyroid
(3) *Corticotrophin* (ACTH) – maintains normal function of the adrenal glands
(4) *Adipokinin* or *lipotropin* – enhances movement of fat from the liver
(5) *Melanocyte stimulating* hormone
(6) *Prolactin* – promotes secretion of milk.

The posterior part hormones are:

(7) *Follicular stimulating* hormones
(8) *Luteinising* hormone.

Bovine somatotrophin (BST)
Somatotrophin was found to stimulate growth and also increase the milk yield in lactating animals. All cows produce natural BST with minute quantities found

in all cow's milk. High yielding dairy cows have been found to have higher levels of natural BST. Technological developments have meant that a recombinant BST has been developed and manufactured in commercial quantities. To be effective it must be injected into the bloodstream as it is broken down in the digestive tract.

BST is legally a medicine and two commercial BSTs have been considered by the Veterinary Products Committee (VPC) for licensing. The VPC considered the scientific evidence and was satisfied that there were no issues of animal health and welfare or problems with milk safety for humans. The EU, however, is still not convinced. At present the commercial BSTs are only authorised for field trials and a moratorium on the marketing and use of BST is in effect until the end of 1999. Recombinant BST is licensed for sale in many other countries including the USA, South Africa, Pakistan, Russia, Romania and Zimbabwe.

Thyroid gland

This consists of two lateral lobes, lying on either side of the trachea close to the larynx, connected inferiorly by a narrow isthmus (1 cm in width). In the bovine each lobe measures $7 \, cm \times 2 \, cm$. It is dark red in colour in the bovine and sheep, and relatively large and chocolate-coloured in the pig. The active principle is *thyroxine*, which has the effect of speeding up metabolism. In young animals it stimulates growth. Deficiency of it produces *cretinism*.

Iodine in the diet is necessary to maintain a normally functioning gland. Deficiency of iodine causes *goitre*, which is an enlargement of the thyroid gland often accompanied by *exophthalmus* or protruding eyes.

Thyroid deficiency (hypothyroidism) causes *myxoedema*, which is characterised by a slowing of physical and mental processes.

Parathyroid glands

These are very small glands, usually four in number. In the bovine they are situated close to the thyroid gland, but in other animals the situations are variable. They secrete *parathormone*, which regulates the metabolism of calcium and phosophorus.

Pancreas

Only part of the pancreas (see p. 58) acts as a ductless gland, i.e. the part made of small conglomerates of cells known as the islets of Langerhans. The rest secretes pancreatic juice, which goes via the pancreatic duct to the small intestine. The β cells of islets of Langerhans produce *insulin*, which controls the level of sugar in the blood. Lack of insulin causes diabetes. The β cells produce the other hormone, *glucagon*, which raises blood sugar levels by stimulating the liver. Glucagon plays an important part during fasting or starvation.

Adrenals or suprarenals

These are paired and are small, elongated glands that lie anterior to the kidneys. In the bovine they measure 5–8 cm. They are composed of a medulla and a cortex. The medulla produces the hormones *adrenaline* and *noradrenaline*, which regulate vascular tone and heart action. Production is increased in time of stress, so that cardiac output is increased and the blood pressure raised. The cortex produces *hydrocortisone, corticosterone* and aldosterone. Production of these is controlled by ACTH from the pituitary. Hydrocortisone and corticosterone regulate the rate of tissue protein breakdown and the utilisation oif carbohydrates and fat. Deficiency of hydrocortisone causes Addison's disease. Aldosterone conserves salt in the body.

Ovaries

These are paired glands that besides producing the ova also produce the oestrogens *oestradiol* and *oestrone*, which control the actions of the female genital and related organs. The corpus luteum produces progesterone which promotes blood supply to the uterus.

Testes

These are also paired glands that besides producing sperm also secrete the male hormone *testosterone*, which regulates the male characteristics.

Placenta

This secretes the hormone *chorionic gonadotrophin*, which helps to maintain pregnancy.

Duodenum

The presence of food stimulates the duodenum to produce the hormone *secretin*, which stimulates the production of the enzymes of the pancreas.

Thymus or sweetbread

This is thought to be a ductless gland but its function is not known. It is thought to have a role in growth processes, antibody formation and sexual maturation. It is pinkish white, is distinctly lobulated and consists of two portions. The thoracic portion, which lies in the thoracic cavity, extends as far as the third rib. It is roughly the shape of the palm of the hand, is rich in fat and is often called the 'heart bread'. The second portion, which is poor in fat, is called the 'neck bread'. It consists of two lobes joined at their bases and extending up the neck on either side of the trachea as far up as the larynx. The lobes diminish in size as they pass up the neck.

In the calf the thymus is at its greatest development at 5–6 weeks and weighs up to 1 kg, but gradual atrophy takes place and by the onset of sexual maturity little of the cervical portion remains.

Pineal gland

This is included although its functions are not yet fully understood. It is a small gland situated in the brain and produces a substance called *melatonin*. This is thought to be concerned with skin pigmentation and may also haved an action on the ovaries and testicles.

Slaughter and Age/Sex Determination

Chapter 12
The Slaughter of Animals

There is evidence of a link between the level of stress in the animal and the meat quality, and therefore animals should be kept and transported in comfortable conditions before they are slaughtered. Following the rigours of transport there should be an adequate period of rest before slaughter and an adequate supply of food and water. Animals should be handled without any unnecessary fuss or noise and they should not be stressed. For cattle and sheep this means a quiet and relaxing environment in the lairage; for pigs water sprays may be used to create a relaxed environment.

Legislation requires that animals should be stunned or rendered unconscious before they are bled. Exemptions are made for Jewish and Muslim slaughter (ritual slaughter).

Stunning

After stunning there are two distinct phases. The first phase is known as the tonic or rigid phase in which the animal falls to the floor and lies still and rigid with its front legs extended and the rear legs retracted towards the body. In the second phase, known as the clonic phase, the animal exhibits uncontrolled convulsions or kicking movements. During both of these phases no rhythmic breathing should be evident.

There are three main methods of stunning an animal:

(1) Mechanical stunning
(2) Electrical stunning
(3) Carbon dioxide (CO_2) stunning.

Mechanical stunning

This method is commonly used on cattle and sheep. Pigs can be stunned by this method; however, this causes excessive convulsions making it difficult to shackle the legs, therefore electrical and CO_2 stunning tends to be used.

There are two types of mechanical stunning device:

(1)   The invasive captive bolt
(2)   The non-invasive captive bolt (knocker).

Both types work by the same principle. A trigger mechanism explodes a blank cartridge, which drives the bolt. It is the velocity of the bolt that is the main factor in providing the required energy for an efficient stun. It is therefore very important that the stunning device be regularly maintained and serviced. The non-invasive or knocker type has a mushroom-shaped end to the bolt. When the bolt hits the skull it stuns the animal. In the invasive type the bolt is driven through the skull into the brain causing invasive damage to the cortex and mid-brain. The animal is rendered incapable of recovery due to the brain damage.

To ensure that the animal is stunned correctly it is very important that the correct site for shooting be used. In cattle this is a point on the forehead at the intersection of two imaginary lines drawn from the base of the horns to the eyes on the opposite side. In sheep and domesticated deer the point is at the highest point of the head at the mid-point between the ears and aimed towards the jaw line. In pigs it is about 2.5 cm above the level of the eyes on the mid-line and at right angles to the forehead. In boars and sows it is 5 cm above the level of the eyes and to one side of the mid-line to avoid the maximum thickness of skull bone.

Pithing

After cattle are stunned, they are sometimes pithed before bleeding. This is done by inserting a long, thin flexible metal rod through the hole in the skull made by the bolt of the pistol. It has the effect of destroying the medulla oblongata and therefore minimising reflex muscular action that takes place during sticking and dressing of the carcass. Bleeding is not affected in any appreciable way.

Pithing rods must be kept clean and disinfected between use on each animal.

Electrical stunning

This consists of passing a 50-Hz electrical current through the brain. This induces a state of immediate epilepsy in the brain during which time the animal is unconscious. The length of time the electrical stun is applied has no effect on the length of the tonic or clonic phases. To ensure a good stun the position of the tongs is crucial. The stun is also dependent on the voltage, the resistance of the animal, the contact area and the pressure applied by the tongs. Some systems will have fail-safe circuitry which passes a low voltage when the tongs are first applied to determine the resistance of the animal. If the resistance measured will allow a stun, then the full voltage will be discharged; if the resistance will not allow a stun, then the full voltage is not discharged.

This type of stunning is mainly used for pigs, sheep and calves. It is not particularly satisfactory for sheep due to the insulating effects of the wool and the positioning of the tongs on horned sheep. Bleeding should commence within 5 seconds of stunning or 'blood splashing' may occur (p. 180).

There are also stun-kill devices which stun the animal and cause cardiac arrest at the same time. One such device is the head to back or cardiac arrest stunner. Used mainly for sheep, the electrical contact is improved by water spraying the sheep before and spraying water over the front head electrodes. Other new types of electrical stunning devices use high frequency (over 300 Hz) voltages with different or hybrid electrical waves.

Carbon dioxide (CO₂) stunning

This method is used commonly for pigs. The pigs are passed through a well with a CO_2 and air atmosphere. Legally a minimum of a 70% concentration of CO_2 by volume is required, but a 90% concentration is recommended. The pigs are rendered unconscious due to the acidification of the cerebrospinal fluid (CSF) upon inhalation of the CO_2. The pH of the CSF drops from its normal level of 7.4 to 6.8. The advantage of this method is that blood splashing is eliminated. It also removes the human element required in the electrical stunning.

Bleeding of the animal (exsanguination) ('sticking')

This is the only procedure that must be assumed to cause the death of the animal: none of the stunning methods can be assumed to have killed the animal. Legally, no other slaughter or dressing procedures should be carried out before the expiry of at least 30 seconds for cattle and 20 seconds for sheep, goats, pigs and deer. Sticking should occur within 15 seconds of stunning.

About 40–60% of the total blood volume is lost during bleeding of the animal. The remainder is largely retained in the viscera. Only about 3–5% remains in the muscles.

Cattle

After the animal has been stunned and pithed, the skin is incised along the jugular furrow with one knife. A second knife is then used to sever the aorta in the thoracic cavity. The knives should be sterilised between each incision.

Bleeding should continue for 5–6 minutes. The average amount of blood obtained from cattle is about 13.5 litres.

Sheep

Sheep are generally stunned either by a captive bolt pistol or by electricity. If a captive bolt pistol is used, the sheep must be stunned separately and not in the sight of other sheep. Bleeding is done by making an incision in the jugular furrow close to the head and severing the carotid arteries. At the same time the head is jerked back to rupture the spinal cord at the base of the skull. This stops reflex muscular action similar to pithing in cattle. Bleeding should last for about 5 minutes and the amount of blood obtained is about 2 litres.

Pigs

In pigs the knife is inserted in the mid-line of the neck in the depression in front of the sternum. The anterior vena cava is then severed at the entrance of the chest. It is important not to puncture the pleura here or back bleeding or oversticking occurs (see p. 181). This is fairly common in pigs because of their short necks. Pigs should be allowed to bleed for about 5 minutes. The amount of blood obtained is from 2 to 4 litres according to size.

Deer

Domesticated deer are bled in the same way as pigs. The amount of blood obtained varies from 2 to 4 litres according to size.

Ritual slaughter

Legislation allows for the slaughter of animals without previous stunning in the (1) Jewish, and (2) Islamic or Muslim methods. The same exemption also applies for the ritual slaughter of poultry. Apart from poultry, only cloven-footed animals that chew the cud are eaten by Jews and Muslims. In their slaughterhouses, therefore, only cattle, sheep and goats are ritually slaughtered.

It has been stated frequently that animals bleed better by the Jewish or Muslim than by other methods, but this is doubtful. There is no scientific evidence that different methods of slaughter have any effect on the efficiency of bleeding.

Jews and Muslims use their own licensed slaughtermen.

Jewish method of slaughter – Shechita

A swift cut is made across the neck with a very sharp knife. This severs the skin, underlying muscles, trachea, oesophagus, jugular veins and carotid arteries.

The five principles of Shechita are that the neck should be cut without pause, pressure, stabbing, slanting or tearing. If the knife receives any nick during the operation the slaughtered animal is considered unfit for Jewish consumption. When the diaphragm is exposed during dressing of the carcass, the shochet or Jewish cutter pierces this and subjects the thoracic organs to a manual examination. This is known as 'searching'. Any adhesions of the lungs found are examined visually and if deemed detrimental to the animal when it was alive, the carcass is pronounced 'terefah' or unfit for Jewish consumption. Carcasses found fit or 'Kosher' must have the meat porged by removal of the blood vessels and sinews. It is for this reason that the forequarters, which are easily porged, are eaten by the Jews. The hindquarters, which are difficult to porge, are seldom eaten by them but are sold to the non-Jewish population who, although they may be opposed to ritual slaughter, may eat such hindquarter meat not knowing that the animal was killed by this method.

Muslim method of slaughter – halāl

This method is similar to the Jewish method but there is no searching or porging after slaughter and both fore-and hindquarters are eaten.

Rigor mortis

After death rigor mortis occurs. It develops 4–8 hours after slaughter in pigs, 8–12 hours after in sheep and 12–24 hours after in cattle.

The pH of the muscle at the time of death is about 7, i.e. neutral. During the process of rigor mortis the glycogen in the muscle turns to lactic acid causing the muscle to become more acid and the pH falls to 5.5–5.8. Owing to the chemical action taking place there is a rise in temperature of about 3°C in the carcass.

The characteristics of rigor mortis are:

(1) Contraction and hardening of muscles
(2) Dullness of muscles through lack of transparency
(3) Stiffness and immobility of joints.

It is associated with the breakdown of adenosine triphosphate (ATP) and its non-replacement because of the lack of oxygen.

Rigor mortis gradually disappears after 24 hours of its onset. Various factors can affect it. The higher the ambient temperature the quicker are its onset and it disappearance. Lower temperatures have the opposite effect. In fevered animals the resulting rigor mortis may be very slight and transient.

A low pH is a desirable factor for the keeping quality and tenderness of meat.

The hardening of fat after death is due to the fall in temperature and not to rigor mortis.

Emergency slaughter
(Fresh Meat (Hygiene and Inspection) Regulations 1995, Regulation 17)

Emergency slaughter of animals is carried out because of either accident or disease. Common causes of emergency slaughter are:

(1) Fractures of limbs or pelvis
(2) Extensive bruising or injuries, e.g. accidents and trampling during transit
(3) Respiratory distress, e.g. in choke or tympanites
(4) Prolonged recumbency, e.g. milk fever
(5) Difficult parturition
(6) Partial asphyxiation – occurring often in pigs during transit
(7) Heat stroke – this also occurs in pigs during transit in hot weather.

It is important to bear in mind the possibility of anthrax in emergency slaughter.

The carcass and offal in any case of emergency slaughter should receive a very thorough inspection and if there is any doubt, samples should be submitted for bacteriological examination.

Lairaging of animals

Every slaughterhouse must have suitable and sufficient lairages as required by Schedule 1(b) of the Fresh Meat (Hygiene and Inspection) Regulations 1995, which must include a lockable pen in which animals, diseased or injured, or suspected of being diseased or injured, may be isolated from other animals.

Animals may not be kept for longer than 72 hours in the lairages before slaughter, unless the Official Veterinary Surgeon (OVS) has given consent due to exceptional circumstances.

Ante-mortem inspection

Animals awaiting slaughter should be inspected before they are slaughtered and this is done in the lairages. It is therefore important that the layout and construction of the lairages should be such that it is easy for the animals to be seen. While the ante-mortem inspection is being carried out, other points should be noticed relating to regulations regarding feeding, watering, bedding, etc.

Any signs of disease, distress, injury, etc. should be noted and the appropriate action taken. Important diseases that may be found at ante-mortem inspection are anthrax, foot and mouth disease, bovine spongiform encephalopathy, sheep scab, mange, orf, swine erysipelas, swine fever and swine vesicular disease.

Schedule 8 of the Fresh Meat (Hygiene and Inspection) Regulations 1995 contains the statutory requirements to be fulfilled during the ante-mortem inspection.

Post-mortem inspection

Under Schedule 10 of the Fresh Meat (Hygiene and Inspection) Regulations 1995 the requirements and methods of undertaking the post-mortem inspection

Table 12.1 Physiological data relating to the various species.

	Temperature °C (°F)	Pulse (per min)	Respiration (per min)	Gestation (days)
Cattle	39 (102)	50	12–16	280
Sheep and goats	39.5 (103)	75	12–20	147
Pigs	39 (102)	75	10–16	112
Horses	38 (100)	36	8–12	340
Deer	38.5 (101)	60–80	13–15	(see p. 7)

of the slaughtered animal are clearly defined. The requirements vary depending on the specific type, age and condition of the animal being inspected.

Line slaughter

Nowadays most animals after slaughter are dressed on the 'line' system. This entails that after stunning (except in the case of the Jewish and Muslim methods) the animals are shackled by a hind leg and lifted by means of either a hoist or an elevator on to an overhead rail before being bled.

In the cases of the small animals, which are generally stunned electrically, this tends to produce rather a lot of 'blood splashing'. The time taken for these animals to be shackled, hoisted and bled is generally around 35–40 seconds. According to the latest experimental figures bleeding should take place within 5 seconds of electrical stunning to prevent 'blood splashing'.

The line system does raise the problem of identifying offals with carcasses unless the offals move along with the carcasses. However, not all lines work on this principle. Once it is realised that there is this problem, a little thought and ingenuity can overcome it. There must be an adequate number of inspectors manning the line to do the necessary 100% inspection required by law.

Electrical stimulation of carcasses

Benefits claimed for this process are:

(1)   Tenderness is increased by up to 30%.
(2)   Flavour is increased by up to 10%.
(3)   Colour of the meat is better by 10%.
(4)   It enables hot boning immediately after slaughter.
(5)   The meat keeps longer and is said to have a shorter cooking time.
(6)   Helps in the bleeding process.
(7)   Prevents cold shortening in lambs.

There are various methods of carrying out the process but probably the best and safest is the one using a low voltage stimulation unit, which is earthed through the overhead rail and its own earth.

Immediately after sticking, a skull probe is inserted into the skull through the hole made by the captive bolt. A charge of 90 volts is applied for about 30 seconds. In cattle the probe passes through the medulla and into the spinal cord.

Hot deboning of carcasses

A very high degree of hygiene is required in this fairly recent innovation. Instead of removing the meat from cold joints the meat is removed from the warm carcass. The muscles are seamed out to a great extent so that there is less drip loss and there is a better colour and shape to the final product. A side of beef can be deboned by one operative in less than 1 hour.

Definitions

Meat is all parts of animals which are suitable for human consumption. This includes all domestic animals of the following species: bovine animals (including buffalo and bison), swine, sheep, goats, solipeds and farmed game.

Carcass or *carcase* is the whole body of one of the above animals (except pigs) that has been slaughtered, after bleeding, evisceration and removal of the limbs at the carpus and tarsus, removal of the head, tail, udder and removal of the skin. The pig carcass still has the skin attached.

Offal is fresh meat other than that of the carcass, whether or not naturally connected to the carcass.

Viscera is the term given to the offal from the thoracic, abdominal and pelvic cavities, including the trachea and oesophagus.

Chapter 13
Sex Characteristics and Estimation of Age

Sex characteristics of carcasses

Cattle

Cow (Fig. 13.1)

(1) Area of udder removal obvious
(2) Supramammary node or part may be left on carcass
(3) Pelvic cavity is wide, pubic bone is thin, almost straught, tubercle is small and not cartilaginous
(4) Gracilis muscle appears bean-shaped
(5) No bulbo-cavernosus muscle or root of penis or inguinal canal
(6) Remains of broad ligaments of uterus
(7) Fat is irregularly distributed and rough and yellow
(8) Bones are small, e.g. carpus.

Heifer

(1) Udder is white, smooth and fatty
(2) No bulbo-cavernosus muscle or root of penis or inguinal canal
(3) Cartilage not ossified, e.g. pubic tubercle, sternum and ends of thoracic vertebral spines
(4) Fat is more evenly distributed, smooth and lighter in colour
(5) Gracilis muscle appears bean-shaped.

Bullock (castrated) males (Fig. 13.1)

(1) Muscles are more developed and bones are larger, e.g. carpus
(2) Scrotal (cod) fat is abundant
(3) Pelvic cavity is narrow, floor is angular and pubic tubercle is large and cartilaginous
(4) Root of penis is present
(5) Marked bulbo-cavernosus muscle

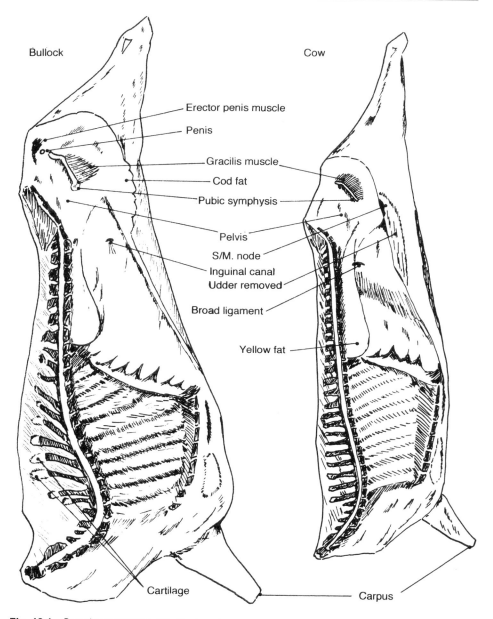

Fig. 13.1 Sex characteristics of bullock and cow.

(6)   Gracilis muscle appears triangular because posterior part is covered with fat
(7)   Internal inguinal ring is obvious and remains of the vessels present.

Bull

(1)   Massive neck and shoulder muscles (crest)
(2)   Dark red colour of muscle and absence of fat
(3)   Open internal and external inguinal rings and no cod fat
(4)   Pelvic cavity is narrow, floor angular and pubic tubercle is large
(5)   Root of penis present and strong bulbo-cavernosus muscle
(6)   Gracilis muscle appears triangular.

Young entire male (young bull)
These are killed at about 18 months. They have a better food conversion rate than bullocks and have less fat. They are more strongly developed than bullocks, especially in the shoulder region. They have more or less the same characteristics as older bulls.

Sheep

Ram or tup

(1)   Strong muscular forequarter
(2)   Open inguinal rings
(3)   Cod fat is sparse or absent
(4)   Root of penis is present

Wether (castrated male) (Fig. 13.2)

(1)   Carcass is usually well proportioned with evenly distributed fat
(2)   Labulated cod fat
(3)   Root of penis is present.

Gimmer (virgin female) (Fig. 13.2)

(1)   Carcass is characterised by its symmetrical shape
(2)   Smooth convex udder is composed mainly of fat.

Ewe

(1)   Carcass is angular in shape with long thin neck and poor legs
(2)   Udder tissue is brown, spongy and never sets. If removed, it leaves roughened area and portions of it and supramammary nodes may remain on carcass.

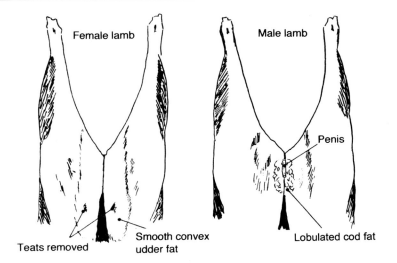

Fig. 13.2 Sex characteristics of female and male lamb.

Differentiation of sheep and goat carcasses

Sheep and goat carcasses are very similar but goat carcasses are very lean and would normally only be confused with poor ewe carcasses. The differences are given in Table 13.1.

Table 13.1 Differences between sheep and goat carcasses.

Ewe	Goat
Lack of kidney fat	Abundant kidney fat
Shorter legs	Longer legs
In unsplit carcasses hind legs form a U-shape	In unsplit carcasses hind legs form a V-shape
Tail is thicker and is tucked in between hind legs	Tail is thinner and falls away from carcass
Barrel-shaped chest	Narrow chest
Subcutaneous tissue is not sticky	Subcutaneous tissue is sticky and hairs tend to adhere

Pigs

Boar

(1) Presence of shield. This is an oval, strongly developed area of cartilage over the shoulder region
(2) Removal of area of scrotum inside thighs
(3) Root of penis is present
(4) Bulbo-cavernosus muscle is present
(5) Protractor muscle of prepuce is present

(6) V-flap in belly incision. This is a flap made in the skin of the abdomen when the prepuce is removed during dressing of the carcass.

Hog (castrated male) (Fig. 13.3)

(1) Root of penis is present.
(2) Castration dip. This is due to contraction of fibrous tissue.
(3) Protractor muscle of prepuce is present in the belly fat, which is convavely grooved.
(4) Gracilis muscle is partially fat covered.
(5) V-flap in belly incision.

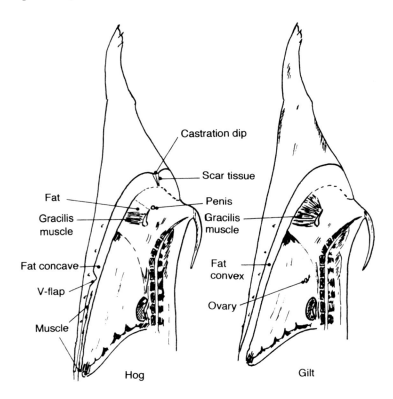

Fig. 13.3 Sex characteristics of pigs.

Young entire male pig (young boar)
This type of pig is becoming more popular as it has a better food conversion rate and has less fat than the castrate. Although the shield is absent, it has the disadvantage of being strongly developed in the shoulder region. The characteristics are the same as the older boar except for the absence of the shield.

Problems have arisen with entire male pigs because they are lean and, in common with other lean pigs, have the following undesirable characteristics:

(1)   Soft fat
(2)   Poor setting of cuts
(3)   Fat and lean separation.

Gilt (virgin female) (Fig. 13.3)

(1)   All male characteristics as above are absent
(2)   Belly incision is straight and fat is convex
(3)   Gracilis muscle appears bean-shaped and is fat free
(4)   Occasionally the ovaries are left in abdomen.

Sow

(1)   Greater development of udders and teats
(2)   Pelvic cavity is wide – generally more than a handsbreadth

Estimation of age

All these indications are approximate.

Cattle

By the teeth

(1)   At birth or soon after, there are eight milk or temporary incisor teeth in lower jaw
(2)   Eruption of permanent incisors:

Centrals	1 year 9 months
Lateral centrals	2 years 3 months
Laterals	2 years 9 months
Corners	3 years 3 months

(3)   Neck of centrals visible at 6 years
Neck of lateral centrals visible at 7 years
Neck of laterals visible at 8 years
Neck of corners visible at 9 years
(4)   Eruption of permanent molars:

4th	6 months
5th	12–18 months
6th	2 years
1st and 2nd	2 years 6 months
3rd	3 years

By the horns
Estimation of the age of cattle by means of the horns entails counting the rings

upon the horns. The first ring appears at about 2 years and one appears every year thereafter, so that age in years in cattle equals the number of rings, plus one.

By the bones
Young animals have cartilage associated with the bones. In the split carcass this is most obvious as the cartilaginous extensions of the spines of the dorsal vertebrae, between the joints of the sternum and the pubic symphysis. The cartilaginous extensions of the dorsal spines are ivory white and are clearly demarcated from the bright red marrow of the dorsal spines. On the first two or three spines the cartilaginous extensions measure up to 5 cm in length, gradually reducing to a few millimetres on the 13th spine. As the animal gets older the cartilage slowly ossifies showing increasing numbers of red islets of bone. At 6 years the cartilages are completely ossified and the junctions with the spines are indistinct. The marrow is also much lighter in colour. The intervertebral and sternal cartilages also give indications of age.

In cows, cartilage is ossified after 3 years. The ischio-pubic symphysis can be cut with a knife up to 3 years. Similarly, the vertebral red bone marrow becomes yellow.

Age of calves
This is estimated by the condition of the hooves, teeth, unbilicus and horns. Newly born calves have soft hooves with conical processes on their solar surfaces. The umbilical stump is grey and moist and firmly attached to the umbilical ring. Cicatrisation of the umbilicus takes place in about 3 weeks and all 8 milk incisor teeth have erupted. By the end of the 3rd week in horned breeds, there is a hard epidermal callosity over the frontal bones. The muscles of immature calves are flabby and greyish red, especially the hind limbs. The marrow is soft and dark red, and the kidney fat is soft and greyish red.

Sheep
(1) At birth or soon after, there are eight milk teeth.
(2) Eruption of permanent incisors:

Centrals	$1-1\frac{1}{2}$ years
Lateral centrals	$1\frac{1}{2}-2$ years
Laterals	$2-2\frac{1}{2}$ years
Corners	3 years
Notch between centrals	6 years

Pigs
Eruption of permanent incisors (not reliable):

Laterals	9 months
Centrals	12–15 months
Inner laterals	16–20 months

Horse

Eruption of the six upper and lower permanent incisors:

Centrals	$2\frac{1}{2}$ years
Laterals	$3\frac{1}{2}$ years
Corners	$4\frac{1}{2}$ years

Deer

The estimation of the age of deer is much more complicated than in the other animals. The lower canine tooth looks like an incisor and for convenience is called the 4th incisor.

(1) Birth to 6 months in lower jaw: 4 milk incisors, 3 milk premolars, 1 permanent molar.
(2) 12–18 months: 1 permanent incisor, 3 milk incisors, 3 milk premolars and 2 permanent molars.
(3) $2\frac{1}{2}$ years: 4 permanent incisors, 3 permanent premolars, 3 permanent molars.

The age of deer up to 10 years can be estimated fairly accurately by an expert by the condition of the 1st permanent molar. The most convenient method, however, is by comparison with mandibles from deer of known ages.

Important note

It is essential that the student, before going on to the next chapters dealing with pathology, specific diseases, etc., should have learned fully the preceding chapters. It cannot be stressed too much that the student must have a complete knowledge of the sex of the carcass and of the specific organ or tissue with which he or she is dealing. It is ridiculous to know all about, for example, a rare condition, such as eosinophilic myositis, and yet not to know the difference between a bullock carcass and a heifer carcass, or the difference between a calf liver and a lamb liver.

Pathology and Judgement in Disease

Judgement is the most difficult part of meat inspection. It is easy to reject meat but not easy to know what to pass as fit for human consumption.

Diseases vary in their severity, extent and spread within the animal body. The acute stage of the disease is always associated with inflammation as the disease is active and progressive, but of course the disease may be of the mild or chronic type. It is obvious that in meat inspection all stages are encountered, from very slight to very severe with all the possible graduations in between.

Schedule 10 of The Fresh Meat (Hygiene and Inspection) Regulations 1995 lists certain diseases and conditions that render the whole carcass and offal as unfit for human consumption. Obviously there is no room for doubt in a disease such as anthrax, but in another condition such as bruising (extensive and severe) the question arises as to what is extensive and what is severe. Since extensive and severe cannot be stated precisely in words, judgement becomes very important, and it can only be decided upon by experience and a sound knowledge of all the factors involved. As a general guide when a disease or condition that could have entered the bloodstream of the animal e.g. septic pleurisy and pneumonia, is identified and caused systemic infection, then the appropriate follow-up inspections should be carried out. These will include inspection of the lymph nodes and kidneys to assess the extent of spread of the disease or condition through the animal and whether it has become systemic or not, e.g. pyaemia and septicaemia. Other diseases or conditions may cause wasting or incapacitation of the animal, for example arthritis or rheumatism, so judgement will be based on any other condition that results from the wasting or incapacitation of that animal, e.g. emaciation or oedema.

Judgements are given throughout this section, however, they are only guides as it is not always possible to give a definite judgement without actually seeing the extent and severity of the condition.

Chapter 14
Abnormal and General Pathological Conditions

Before describing the pathological changes brought about by specific diseases it is important to consider certain general physiological and pathological changes.

Where possible it is suggested that books with coloured illustrations of diseases should be used in conjunction with these notes.

Poorness

This is a physiological state that occurs most frequently in very young and older animals, particularly calves, cows, ewes, deer and sows. It can be caused by shortage of food, overmilking, etc. A striking example of poorness due to lack of food occurs in deer in the wild in the winter time. Many deer may die in a severe winter and the condition is known as 'winter death syndrome'. Many deer carcasses in January and February are in poor condition, especially those of hinds that are still in milk. The carcass sets well but there is a marked scarcity of fat, which, however, is of the normal firm consistency. The flesh is generally darker in colour and on the cut surface is firm and dry. If the carcass is allowed to hang for some time, it becomes very dry and dark on the surface.

Judgement: Such carcasses are fit for human consumption and because the meat is tough, are often used for manufacturing purposes, e.g. sausages and cooked meats.

In case of doubt it is advisable to hang the carcass for 12–24 hours before making a judgement.

Emaciation

This condition, in comparison with poorness with which it should not be confused, is due to some pathological condition, generally chronic, e.g. Jöhne's disease in cattle and parasitic infestion in sheep. It is characterised by wasting of muscular tissue and by a reduction in the amount of fat, which is soft, wet and, in advanced cases, gelatinous. The flesh is wet, soft and flabby. This is best detected on a freshly cut surface when the muscles pit on pressure and are soft and sticky to the touch. The carcass does not set and the outside is wet, as are the pleura and peritoneum. The region of the brisket is generally a particularly wet area in cattle. In ewes the kidney fat gives a good indication. Where a doubt exists, the carcass should be hung for 12–24 hours to see if it will set and dry out. Emaciated carcasses in fact tend to get wetter.

Judgement: Total rejection.

Oedema or dropsy

In this condition there is an excessive accumulation of a clear fluid (very similar to lymph) in the tissues or serous sacs of the body [see Plate 1(a)]. According to the sites of the oedema other terms are used:

(1) *Anasarca* when the skin and subcutaneous tissues are affected.
(2) *Hydropericardium, hydrothorax* and *ascites* when there is accumulation of fluid in the pericardium, pleural and peritoneal cavities, respectively.

Oedema may be local or generalised. Local oedema may be due to obstruction of a vein or around an inflammatory area, when it is known as inflammatory oedema. Generalised oedema occurs in cardiac and renal diseases and in chronic wasting diseases, e.g. tuberculosis, Jöhne's disease and parasitic diseases.

In meat inspection many carcasses are rejected for oedema and emaciation.

Judgement: If generalised, total rejection.

Imperfect bleeding (insufficiency of bleeding)

This occurs when the animal is moribund (dying) or very distressed and is said to have been killed to 'save its life'. The flesh is dark, there is capillary bleeding, the organs, particularly liver, lungs and kidneys, are dark and congested and when cut, blood runs out. The intercostal veins are full of blood and are clearly visible. The forelegs often tend to be 'tucked up'. The carcass sets badly and decomposes rapidly.

Judgement: Such carcasses are rejected as unfit for human consumption.

Bruising

Judgement: Dependent on the extent and severity of the bruising. If there is extensive and severe bruising, total rejection, otherwise reject the affected parts.

Haematoma

This is a solid swelling of clotted blood within tissue which has been caused by some physical injury.
   Judgement: Reject the affected parts.

Suffocation

This may result from choking, drowning or trampling and crushing during transit. It is probably the commonest cause of animals arriving dead at the abattoir, particularly in sheep and pigs. In cold weather, pigs huddle together with the result that the one at the bottom of the heap gets suffocated. Blood or bloody froth often emanates from the nostrils. The organs of a suffocated animal are generally congested, especially the lungs, which also contain frothy mucus. The right side of the heart is full of clotted blood and the left side is empty. The flesh is dark and sets badly. The blood vessels, particularly the subcutaneous vessels of the side on which the animal was lying, are markedly congested. The carcass decomposes quickly.
   Judgement: NB   Dead animals should not be eviscerated. Total rejection.

Fevered flesh

This generally arises through the action of bacteria or viruses and their toxins circulating in the blood. The flesh is darker in colour with small, scattered hae-morrhages. The pleura, peritoneum and fat show a diffuse redness and the organs and lymph nodes are congested. The carcass as a whole has a dull red appearance and can be easily picked out if alongside normal carcasses.
   Judgement: Total rejection.

Fetal flesh

This is the flesh of unborn or still-born animals and is regarded as unfit for human consumption. The lungs are solid and sink in water. There is an open urachus (the canal that joins the bladder with the allantoic cavity, which some-times persists after birth, the urine escaping via the umbilicus). The umbilical veins and arteries gape widely. The eyes may be closed and the hooves are soft and unwalked upon ('golden slippers'). Further signs are the flabby, sodden conditions of the muscles, the gelatinous condition of the connective tissue around the kidneys and the presence of red marrow in the long bones. The sto-mach is empty.
   Judgement: Total rejection.

Immaturity

The only food animal that is likely to be sold for food while immature is the calf. The Fresh Meat (Hygiene and Inspection) Regulations 1995, Schedule 10, state:

> ... any immature carcass which is oedematous or in poor physical condition, together with any offal or blood is unfit for human consumption.

This of course is not a great help as one still has to decide what an immature carcass is. Various countries have regulations that calves shall not be less than so many days old, but unless the date of birth is known, this is no great help. Other countries go by the weight, but as the size of calves varies with the different breeds, this does not seem very sensible either.

The following is probably the best guide:

(1)   the meat has the appearance of being water-soaked, is loose, flabby and tears easily and can be perforated by the fingers, or
(2)   the colour is greyish-red, or
(3)   good muscular development especially of the hind legs is lacking,
(4)   tissue around the kidneys is oedematous, dirty yellow or greyish red, tough and intermixed with islands of fat.

Judgement: Total rejection.

Abnormal odours

Abnormal odours, especially the male sexual odour, are most apparent immediately after slaughter. They may result from:

(1)   Diet, e.g. fish meals.
(2)   Drugs administered shortly before slaughter, e.g. linseed oil, turpentine, ether, chloroform, aromatic spirits of ammonia, etc.
(3)   Absorption of the odour of strong-smelling substances whilst meat is stored, e.g. refrigerated meat during transport can absorb various smells such as the odour of over-ripe oranges or citrus fruit.
(4)   Catty odours may be found in meat owing to the presence of mesityl oxide. This is a trace impurity in paint thinners and solvents, in lacquers, adhesives, flooring compounds and plastic wrapping materials.
(5)   Sexual odour. This is principally noticed in mature boars and male deers in rut and is due to the presence of a steroid, androstenone, in the fat. Boar salivary glands when boiled in water give off a musty smell. The flesh of buck goats may also have an unpleasant smell similar to that from their skin and is probably conveyed by hand during skinning. Newly calved cows or cows heavy in calf may smell of fetal fluids.

(6)   Acetonaemia or ketosis. This is a metabolic disease occurring in cows shortly after calving. Flesh of cows slaughtered while suffering from acetonaemia has a peculiar sweet smell owing to the presence of acetone in the tissues. It is most easily detected from the freshly cut surface. Some people can detect this odour much more easily than others. The odour remains even after cooking, and advantage is taken of this as a method in detecting doubtful cases using a small portion of muscle. The liver may be fatty with a strong smell of acetone.

Rothera's test for acetone
Reagent: 100 g ammonium sulphate; 50 g anhydrous sodium carbonate; 3 g sodium nitroprusside.
   Shake up 10 g of meat in a test-tube containing 15 ml water. Add one teaspoonful of the reagent. Shake and allow to stand for 2–3 minutes. A purple colour denotes the presence of acetone.

(7)   Specific disease, e.g. blackquarter (p. 118), which causes a cheesy smell.
(8)   Abscesses. Those in pigs have a particularly nasty smell, especially if fat is affected (p. 104).
(9)   Gangrene (p. 112).
(10)   Putrefaction.

Judgement: All cases of abnormal odours, including sexual odours, when pronounced are totally rejected as most odours become more pronounced on cooking. The method generally used for testing odours is to take a piece of meat 24 hours after slaughter and either boil in water or fry.

(11)   Bone taint. This is associated with the growth of the putrefactive anaerobic bacteria *Clostridium perfringens* and *Cl. putrefaciens*, giving a very typical smell to the musculature. The muscle may retain its normal colour but may change to grey, green and almost black. It generally occurs in the region of the hip joint in large hindquarters. It is common in imported hindquarters, but also occurs in home-killed cattle. The cause is not known, but various theories have been put forward, e.g. infection via the sticking knife and exhaustion of animals before slaughter. However, the main cause is probably improper cooling of the carcass, especially in hot, sultry weather. The putrefaction is said to start in the marrow or synovial fluid. Bone taint is a local condition requiring rejection of affected parts although the condition may spread quite extensively, and it is a matter of trimming until unaffected muscle is reached.
   NB   Bone marrow and synovial fluid, which are neutral in reaction (pH 7.0), are ideal situations for the growth of anaerobic bacteria.

Judgement: Reject affected tissues.

Inflammation

This is a defence mechanism of the body and is the series of changes that take place in living tissue as the result of an injury that has not been sufficient to cause the death of the tissue.

Injury may be caused by bacteria or their toxins, parasites, chemicals, heat or cold, or mechanical damage. The changes are (1) heat, (2) pain, (3) redness, (4) swelling and (5) disturbance of function.

When a tissue is injured, there is first dilatation of arterioles and capillaries leading to heat and redness. This is followed by swelling of the cells of the capillary walls, causing the flow of blood to slow down. Because of the damaged capillary walls an abnormal amount of lymph enters the tissues causing swelling, and leucocytes that possess the power of amoeboid movement now migrate through and are attracted to the inflamed area. The accumulation of leucocytes, which if excessive produces pus, is part of the defensive mechanism of the body, as the leucocytes have the power of absorbing and digesting bacteria, etc. Inflammation may be either acute or chronic.

An *abscess* is a collection of pus enclosed in a fibrous capsule.

Judgement: Abscesses are a visual sign of infection. Secondary inspection for pyaemia, septicaemia, viraemia and toxaemia should be carried out. If evidence of systemic infection is found, then total rejection, otherwise reject affected parts.

Machine damage

Pigs are normally scalded at 60°C (140°F) for 1–2 minutes. If the water temperature is too high or immersion too long, the skin and subcutaneous fat become semi-cooked and soft. The result is that the beaters of the dehairing machine loosen or tear the skin and the subcutaneous fat becomes soft and mushy. Hairs adhere to the exposed fat and muscle and extensive trimming of the skin and muscles may be necessary.

Joints of the legs can be dislocated in the dehairing machine but there is no bruising or bleeding as the pigs have already been bled.

Faecal contamination

This is the physical contamination of the carcass or organs by stomach or intestinal contents. It is caused by damage to the stomach or intestinal tract during the slaughter and dressing of the animal. This type of contamination is a significant route of transmission for food poisoning organisms such as *Campylobacter* (p. 225), *Salmonella* (P. 226) and *Escherichia coli* (p. 228).

Judgement: Trim and reject the affected parts.

Pigmentation

Abnormal colour or abnormal positioning of colour is occasionally found in animal tissues.

Anthracosis

Black or bluish black pigmentation of lymph nodes of lungs, particularly the bronchials, and of the lung substance due to the inhalation of coal dust. The mesenteric lymph nodes may also be affected by ingestion.

Judgement: Reject affected parts.

Bile staining

This is a yellowish green pigmentation that may be found on the surface of the carcass or organs. It is due to staining by bile. Bile may be released from the gall bladder during evisceration.

Judgement: Trim and reject the affected parts.

Brown atrophy (lipofuchsinosis)

This condition is associated with ageing, especially when accompanied by a chronic wasting disease. The colour is due to a brownish pigment and can occur in any tissue but is probably most pronounced in the hearts of old cows.

Judgement: Fit.

Brine staining

This is a pale greenish colour found on the surfaces of imported carcasses and is due to leakage of brine or calcium chloride from the refrigeration plant. The staining may penetrate the muscular tissue, which becomes darkened and has a salty or bitter taste.

Judgement: Depends upon severity of the condition.

Carotene pigmentation

This is confined solely to fat and is seen in Jersey and Guernsey cattle; it is commonly seen in old cows of other breeds and dows. The yellow colour of Channel Islands milk is due to carotene pigmentation of the butter fat.

Judgement: Fit.

Rimmington and Fowrie test

This is a simple and accurate way of differentiating between jaundice and carotene. Place 2 g of fat in a test tube and add 5 ml of a 5% solution of sodium hydroxide. Boil for about 1 minute, shaking frequently until the fat is dissolved. Then cool under tap until tube is comfortably warm to the hand. Add an equal volume of ether and mix gently. Allow to settle. The solution settles out into two layers. The bile salts are soluble in water and so if colour is due to jaundice, the bottom layer is coloured yellow. If colour is due to carotene or xanthophylls, the top layer is coloured yellow, as these are souble in ether. Judgement is easier if the test tube is viewed against a white background. Carotene pigmentation is not a reason for rejection.

Dark cutting beef or dark firm and dry pork (DFD)

Both describe the same condition, as does 'glazy bacon'.

These are caused by a high pH of the muscle at slaughter [cf. PSE (p. 108) of pork]. If the pH is between 5.8 and 7, the muscle gets progressively darker in colour. The high pH arises because most of the glycogen in the muscle before death had been used. It is associated with prolonged or chronic stress.

Chilling and lack of feed tend to increase the incidence, and it is more prevalent in frosty weather. The meat is palatable and provides the same nutritive values as normal beef.

It has been a particular problem in 'bull beef' production.

As the pH is high the surviving activity of the cytochrome enzymes will be greater. Also the muscle proteins will be above their isoelectric point (pH 5.5), i.e. the point at which muscles will lose their associated water, and the muscle fibres will be tightly packed together, presenting a barrier to diffusion. As a result of these factors, the bright red oxymyoglobin is small in amount and the purplish red colour of myoglobin will predominate. Furthermore, the high ultimate pH alters the absorption characteristics of the myoglobin and the meat surfaces become a darker red. Such meat will also appear dark because its surface does not scatter light to the same extent as will the more open surface of meat of lower ultimate pH.

Judgement: Depends upon the severity of the condition.

Eosinophilic myositis

This is a rare condition, showing light green patches and streaks in muscular tissue of cattle, sheep, pigs and horses. The cause is unknown.

Judgement: Reject affected parts.

Freezer burn

This is described on p. 206.

Injection coloration

Occasionally subcutaneous tissues, lymph nodes, fat and muscle may be found to be coloured, owing to the injection of coloured medical products. Always examine the associated lymph nodes.

Judgement: Reject affected parts.

Jaundice or icterus

In this condition the tissues of the body are coloured yellow. This is most obvious in the white tissues of the body, e.g. fat, skin of pigs, spinal cord and meninges, tendon sheaths and white of the eye. The coloration is due to the deposition of bile pigments that have been absorbed into the bloodstream. This can be brought about by various conditions, for example:

(1)   cirrhosis of the liver (particularly in pigs)
(2)   blockage of the bile ducts by either calculi, tumours or parasites
(3)   specific diseases in which there is increased destruction of blood corpuscles by infective organisms, e.g. leptospirosis in pigs and red-water in cattle.

The condition varies from slight to very severe, and carcasses and offal should be rejected. It is important to inspect jaundiced carcasses in daylight, as the condition is difficult to see in artificial light.

It is also important to differentiate jaundice from pigmentation due to carotene or xanthophylls. (See Rimmington and Fowrie test on p. 105.)

Judgement: Total rejection.

Melanosis

This is a condition in which the black pigment melanin, which normally colours hair, horns, eyes, etc., is found in abnormal positions in the body. It is found most often in calves, but can occur in any animal except albinos. There is little doubt that the condition is congenital and that the pigment is deposited in early fetal life. Melanotic tumours are found, particularly, in grey horses.

In the ox, melanosis is most often found affecting the periosteum, particularly of the head bones and ribs, the spinal cord, blood vessels of the hind quarter and the liver and lungs, in which organs it resembles splashes of Indian ink [plate 5(a)].

In the pig, it is commonly found in the black breeds or cross black breeds in the belly fat or mammary tissue of females, when it is called 'seedy cut' or 'seedy belly'. Very occasionally it is found in the belly fat of male pigs.

Judgement: Depending upon the severity of the condition reject affected parts.

Nitrate or nitrite poisoning

This causes a brown colour in carcasses. Up to 83% of the haemoglobin may be in the form of methaemoglobin.
Judgement: Carcasses and offal are rejected.

Ochronosis

This is an extremely rare condition affecting cattle. It is caused by a yellowish brown or chocolate-coloured pigment. It involves cartilage, tendon sheaths and joints. It is sometimes generalised.
Judgement: Total rejection if generalised.

Osteohaematochromatosis

This is also rare and affects calves and pigs. All the bones of the body have a dark brown colour caused by the pigment haematoporphyrin. The teeth, lungs, kidneys and lymph nodes may be affected.
Judgement: Total rejection.

Phosphorescence

The non-pathogenic bacterium *Pseudomonas fluorescens* can grow on the surface of meat causing small luminous areas which glow in the dark. Meat is generally infected in cold rooms in which fish have been stored, as the organism is associated with salt-water fish.
Judgement: Reject surface trimmings.

PSE (pale soft exudate)

This condition occurs in some pigs that have been subjected to severe or acute stress just before slaughter. The pH falls rapidly to 4.7 in affected muscles. Because of the denaturation of the muscle proteins, resulting from the high temperature and increased acidity, the muscle is pale and soft and exudes fluid from any cut surface.

The condition is commoner in some breeds of pigs, e.g. in the Belgian Pietrain.

Affected pork is not unfit for human consumption. After cooking it is drier than normal and has lost some of its flavour. It is unsuitable for curing.
Judgement: Fit.

Xanthosis or xanthomatosis

This is characterised by a brown coloration due to a breakdown pigment of the body, xanthine. It is most commonly found in cattle, affecting striated muscles, particularly the muscles of mastication, heart, kidneys and tongue. In all such cases the adrenal bodies are enlarged and dark brown in colour. The cause is unknown.

It is found most commonly in the Ayrshire breed of cattle and a genetic factor is thought to be involved.

Judgement: Reject affected parts.

'Yellow-fatted' sheep

Most sheep have white fat but a small number have yellow fat. This is due to the deposition of xanthophylls, which are pigments of grass. This also occurs in 'yellow-fatted' rabbits. Normal sheep are able to break down carotene and xanthophylls but 'yellow-fatted' sheep are only able to break down carotene, with the result that the xanthophylls are absorbed into the bloodstream and are deposited in the fatty tissues giving rise to the yellow colour. The inability to break down xanthophylls may be genetic in origin.

The method of differentiating between jaundice and carotene (see p. 105) is also applicable for differentiating between jaundice and xanthophyll coloration.

Judgement: Fit.

Disease

Disease may be defined as deviation from health, i.e. derangement in the structure or the function of any organ or tissue in the animal body. The causes of disease are as follows:

(1) Diet, i.e. insufficient or improper food supply, e.g. rickets when diet is lacking in vitamin D.
(2) Overwork or overstrain, e.g. heart disease.
(3) Trauma or injury, e.g. bruises, fractures, burns, traumatic pericarditis, etc.
(4) Micro-organisms, i.e. bacteria, viruses and protozoa.
(5) Parasites, e.g. worms, mites, ticks, etc.
(6) Poisons or toxins.

The diseases caused by micro-organisms and parasites are the most important in meat inspection.

Micro-organisms

Bacteriology or microbiology is the science of micro-organisms.

Pathogenic bacteria are those that have the power of producing disease.

Commensals are bacteria that occur on the skin or in the body of animals, e.g.

mouth, throat, intestine, without causing any harmful effect. However, various commensals may, under certain circumstances, become pathogenic, and some pathogenic bacteria may become commensals, e.g. in so-called 'carrier' animals.

Micro-organisms are generally classified as follows:

(1) Bacteria – organisms of microscopic size, generally unicellular, though they may be attached to each other to form chains (streptococci), filaments or other aggregates (staphylococci). They usually multiply with great rapidity by binary fission. They are usually spheroidal or cylindrical (cocci) or rod-shaped (bacilli).

Some bacteria may develop a resting phase in the form of 'spores', which are generally resistant. Other forms are motile and possess flagella.

(2) Viruses – organisms of ultramicroscopic size, which can generally only be seen by using an electron microscope, e.g. virus of foot and mouth disease.

(3) Rickettsiae – organisms that are intermediate between bacteria and viruses, e.g. *Coxiella burnetti*, which causes 'Q' fever.

(4) Fungi.

(a) Mould forms – branching filaments (*hyphae*) that interlace and form a meshwork (*mycelium*). They are more highly developed than bacteria, being multicellular, and usually reproduce by means of spores.

(b) Yeast forms – round, oval or elongated units, generally larger than bacteria, Multiply by 'budding'.

(5) Protozoa – regarded as the lowest form of animal life. Protozoal infections are most common in tropical and sub-tropical countries.

(6) Prion – this is thought to be a 'rogue' protein. It has been implicated in the cause of BSE (p. 119). It is even smaller than a virus and is believed to be indestructible.

Infection

Infection is said to occur when the tissues are invaded by living organisms, e.g. bacteria, viruses and parasites, and pathological changes take place.

Paths of infection

In the great majority of cases, the infecting organisms reach the body by (1) direct contact; but the vast majority reach the body via (2) inspired air (i.e. by inspiration) and (3) ingested food or drink (i.e. by ingestion).

This applies to nearly all bacterial and viral infections and to many infections caused by metazoan parasites. In a smaller but very important group, the organisms are introduced by the bite of an animal (inoculation), e.g. rabies, or by the bite of an insect, e.g. myxomatosis.

The first lesion, or morbid change, caused by a disease-producing organism is called the *primary* lesion. This primary lesion is very important in practical meat inspection. As has just been stated, the vast majority of infections reach the body by inspiration or ingestion. Therefore the primary lesions should be found in the respiratory or digestive tracts and that is why it is so important to examine all the offal in routine inspection, as all the offal comes from, or is associated with, the respiratory and digestive tracts.

Bacteraemia

When a small number of organisms enter the bloodstream from a lesion and are spread to various parts of the body, the condition is called a bacteraemia. This is generally only a temporary condition.

Septicaemia

This is a much more serious condition than a bacteraemia. It occurs when bacteria gain a foothold and multiply in the bloodstream. This can be identified by finding petechial haemorrhages in the kidneys [see Plate 3(a)].
   Judgement: Total rejection.

Pyaemia

When pyogenic organisms (i.e. pus-producing organisms) enter the bloodstream and form multiple abscesses throughout the body, the condition is called pyaemia. Pyaemic abscesses are most often found in the lungs, kidneys and liver [plate 5(b)].
   'Tick pyaemia' is a type of pyaemia occurring in lambs following suppurative lesions caused by the secondary effects of tick attacks. The commonest tick is *Ixodes ricinus*.
   Judgement: Total rejection.

Toxaemia

This refers to the circulation in the bloodstream of toxins produced by bacteria. This occurs in all infectious diseases and the illness is often caused by the toxins and not by the presence of the bacteria.
   Judgement: Depends upon the severity of the condition.

Viraemia

This is when viruses enter the bloodstream. The symptoms are similar to those of septicaemia.
   Judgement: Total rejection.

Necrosis

This is death of a tissue or of an organ or part of an organ whilst still in the animal body.

Judgement: Reject affected part.

Caseation

This is a type of negrosis in which the necrotic areas look like cheese. Caseous material has an affinity for salts of lime and this finally becomes calcified and hard, e.g. tuberculous lesions.

Judgement: Reject affected part.

Metaplasia

This is a change from one type of cell into another generally of a simpler type, e.g. steatosis. Another example is the plates of bone found in the 'leaf' fat of pigs probably as the result of spaying or castration.

Judgement: Reject affected part.

Gangrene

The term gangrene is applied when a ncrotic tissue becomes invaded by putre-factive bacteria. It occurs most frequently in tissues liable to contamination, i.e. those tissues in contact with the exterior, for example skin, lungs, intestine, vagina and uterus and in those tissues implicated in penetrating wounds. As gangrene progresses, the tissues become livid, purplish or greenish and then brownish black. It is often accompanied by emphysema and a foul odour.

Judgement: Total rejection if evidence of toxaemia. Reject affected parts if gangrene is localised.

Sapraemia

This is a term seldom used now. It is a condition in which saprophytic bacteria gain access to necrotic tissue within the body, multiply and produce waste products that are absorbed into the blood system and so cause disturbances. Such necrotic tissue may be an abscess in lung or liver or necrotic fetal membranes in the uterus.

Saprophytic bacteria are so called because they live and multiply in the animal body but are incapable of invading healthy tissue and producing disease.

Judgement: Reject affected parts.

Production of toxins

In infection there is another important factor in addition to multiplication and spread of organisms throughout the body. This is the production of poisons or toxins by the organisms. Some bacteria produce very powerful toxins, e.g. in diseases such as tetanus and botulism.

Immunity

When an animal is insusceptible to infection by a given organism it is said to possess an immunity against it. The term is similarly used in relation to the action of toxins. In the case of all organisms and all toxins, some animals are found to be susceptible whilst others are immune. The latter are said to have a natural immunity against the particular organism or toxin.

In an animal susceptible to a disease, immunity may become developed, i.e. acquired immunity.

Active immunity

When an animal has the power to produce its own antibodies or antitoxins, this is known as active immunity. This is the basis of vaccination, i.e. a weakened or dead strain of the organism is introduced into the body. This does not produce disease but the body reacts and produces antibodies or antitoxins and the body is thus taught and is able to produce those antibodies or antitoxins when necessary.

Passive immunity

This is the immunity produced when antibodies or antitoxins are injected into the body in the serum from another animal. Passive immunity is conferred at once, whereas active immunity may take 2 or 3 weeks to develop. However, passive immunity only lasts 2–3 weeks, whereas active immunity lasts for years or even a lifetime.

Hydrogen-ion concentration or pH

The pH of a solution is the measurement of the acidity or alkalinity.

Water or H_2O, or more properly H^+ and OH^-, is neutral. The H^+ or hydrogen ion is acid, whilst the OH^- or hydrozyl ion is alkaline. As there is one of each they cancel each other out and water is therefore neutral.

The pH of water is 7. This is neutral: acid solutions have a pH ranging from 0 to 7, and alkaline solutions over 7.

The pH is generally measured by colour changes in certain dyes, e.g. phenol red goes through various changes from yellow to red between pH 6.8 and 8.4 and nitrazene yellow gives indications between pH 6 and 7.

Electrical instruments known as pH meters are now being used for the PH measurement of meat. This measurement is of value as it gives an indication of the keeping quality of meat.

Meat from cattle just killed is either slightly acid or slightly alkaline: pH 6.5–7.2. During rigor mortis glycogen is changed to lactic acid and it is this acid that causes the pH of muscle to fall rapidly to about 5.6 in 48 hours. This acid state largely prevents the growth of putrefactive bacteria and therefore rapid decomposition. After 48 hours the pH remains static for a while depending to a large extent upon the storage conditions, i.e. temperature, etc. When the pH rises to to 6.4, decomposition is about to start, and when it reaches 6.8 this becomes apparent, e.g. smell, texture and colour ('going green').

Measurement of the pH of meat is sometimes of value in the judgement of borderline cases, especially in cases of:

(1)   febrile disease (fever)
(2)   emergency slaughter
(3)   exhaustion.

This is so because in all these cases there is an excessive use of glycogen before slaughter, with the result that the amount of this is decreased in the muscles and so there is less to be changed into lactic acid.

Chapter 15
Specific Diseases

Specific diseases are those caused by specific organisms, e.g. swine fever is caused by a specific virus, as opposed to other conditions such as pneumonia which can be caused by numerous types of organisms.

Actinobacillosis

This is a disease mainly of cattle caused by *Actinobacillus lignieresi*. It typically affects soft tissues and usually involves, by lympatic spread, the regional lymph nodes. In cattle the tongue is commonly affected [see plate 1(c)]. The typical lesions are small nodules about 1 cm in diameter. These are easily seen and palpated on the lateral surfaces and dorsum of the tongue. Some of the nodules may erode through the surface causing ulcers. In the chronic form there is a marked development of fibrous tissue, which causes enlargement and hardening of the tongue – the typical 'wooden tongue'. Lymph nodes of the head are the commonest sites of infection and not the tongue as is commonly supposed. The gums, soft and hard palates and the muzzle are the other sites. Ulcers of actinobacillosis may be confused with foot and mouth disease ulcers. Less commonly affected are the masseter muscles, reticulum, lungs, liver, pleura and peritoneum. In the mouth the ulcers have sharp edges and granulation tissue bases. In older lesions the edges are rounded and indurated. A typical bright yellow or orange pus is often associated with actinobacillous nodules. This pus is a brighter yellow than tubercular pus and is granular. Also, on cross-section, the nodules tend to protrude as opposed to a tuberculous lesion, which is level and smooth if it is not calcified. As it is sometimes difficult to differentiate between the lesions of actinobacillosis and tuberculosis with the naked eye, microscopic examination is necessary. When the reticulum is affected there is a fibrous thickening of the reticular wall. An abundance of a white, glistening, fibrous tissue is typical of chronic actinobnacillosis. This is particularly noticeable in chronic actinobacillosis of the liver. Unlike lesions of tuberculosis, actinobacillous lesions do not calcify.

In sheep, actinobacillosis is characterised by thickening of the skin of the head and abscesses in the lymph nodes of the head and neck. However, the disease is rare in sheep.

Judgement: Affected organs are rejected. If generalised, carcass and offal are rejected.

Actinomycosis

Actinomycosis is a disease of cattle commonly known as 'lumpy jaw'. It is caused by *Actinomyces bovis*. The lesion is an osteomyelitis, which affects the bones of the lower jaw. The upper jaw is seldom affected. The bone is thickened and enlarged and on cross-section has a honeycomb appearance, showing small abscesses and suppurative tracts. Fistulae may lead to the surrounding tissues discharging into the mouth or on to the skin of the jaw. Lesions do not occur in the regional lymph nodes although they may be enlarged and indurated.

Actinomycosis affects sheep and deer more rarely.

There is a condition called actinomycosis of the sow's udder which shows induration of the udder with thick-walled abscesses. Some are said to be caused by *Actinomyces israelli* or *A. suis* and some by staphylococci.

Judgement: Reject affected parts.

Anthrax

Anthrax is a notifiable disease. It is caused by *Bacillus anthracis*, which is a square-ended rod that occurs in the body fluids singly or in short chains. It is capsulated in the body fluids. Under favourable conditions outside the body it sporulates forming a resistant spore.

Anthrax is primarily a disease of animals, and man is infected secondarily. Any animal may become infected, but well over 90% of approximately 200 confirmed cases in Great Britain each year occur in cattle and about 3% in pigs. Cases have been reported in zoos, in carnivores especially, although there was a case at Chester Zoo in which elephants died through eating contaminated hay.

Humans usually contract anthrax by inoculation through a skin wound ('malignant pustule'), or by inhalation ('woolsorters' disease'). The death rate in humans was about 25% of cases but this has been reduced greatly since the advent of antibiotics. The last human death in Britain from anthrax was in 1974.

The Hebridean island of Gruinard was used as a germ warfare experiment site between 1939 and 1945. Porton Down scientists in 1941 conducted tests involving anthrax spores on sheep. The island has since been uninhabited and no visitors have been allowed because of the danger of contracting anthrax. Treatment of the soil with formaldehyde and sea-water was carried out in 1986. In 1989, 40 sheep were grazed throughout the summer as a trial. The only person allowed on the island is the farmer. The island will remain uninhabited and no visitors will be allowed. Tests have shown that the spores are still viable after more than 50 years, but now only a very small area of the land is still contaminated.

Infection in farm animals usually occurs by the ingestion of anthrax spores in foreign feedingstuffs, or in soil, hay, etc. from pastures after a previous death of an animal from anthrax. Spores can also be carried into rivers in the effluent from knacker's yards and tan yards.

In animals the disease generally runs a rapid course, associated with a high body temperature of up to 42°C (107°F). Death usually occurs within 48 hours of the onset of the illness. Animals are often found dead without any symptoms having been noticed. For this reason any animal that dies suddenly or is found dead should be treated as a suspected anthrax case, as are all animals arriving dead at an abattoir, or found dead or dying in lairages.

Diagnosis is by microscopic examination of a stained-blood, peritoneal or tissue fluid smear. The blood is usually taken from vessels at the base of the ear or undersurface of the tail close to the anus.

The post-mortem picture in the bovine is that of a septicaemia:

(1) Blood may exude from the natural body orifices
(2) Blood is dark and tarry and does not clot readily
(3) Extensive petechiae and ecchymoses of mucous membranes
(4) Liver and kidneys pale and friable
(5) Spleen grossly enlarged and dark
(6) Oedema and blood clots in mesentery, and lymph nodes are haemorrhagic and oedematous
(7) Peritonitis may be present with oedematous fluid in the peritoneal cavity.

The lesions are similar in deer.

In the pig the spleen is seldom enlarged although one or more circumscribed dark nodules may be present in the splenic substance. There may also be oedematous swelling of the neck and submaxillary region. In primary intestinal anthrax in pigs there is focal or multifocal haemorrhagic enteritis. The adjacent peritoneum and mesentery are thickened, oedematous and yellowish with spots and streaks of haemorrhage. the mesenteric lesions extend only as far as the regional lymph nodes, which show haemorrhagic lymphadenitis.

The carcass and offal are rejected and burned.

The carcass of an animal that has died suddenly or is found dead should be left severely alone until a blood, peritoneal or tissue fluid smear has been examined and found to be negative.

Nowadays there is a greater risk of anthrax-infected animals coming into an abattoir because of antibiotic therapy. This can mask the symptoms and may keep an animal alive long enough for it to be sent into an abattoir for slaughter.

If anthrax is suspected or found, the Divisional Veterinary Officer of the Ministry of Agriculture, Fisheries and Food should be notified immediately, so that it can be officially confirmed or otherwise. If positive, suitable measures are put into operation for disinfection of premises and disposal of the carcass – either by burning or burying at least 2 metres from the surface with layers of 30 cm of lime above and below the carcass.

It is essential in an anthrax case that as little blood as possible is spilled. For this reason the nose, vulva and anus of the carcass are generally plugged with cotton wool or tow.

Very thorough disinfection of premises and utensils must be carried out. A hot

5% solution of sodium hydroxide is commonly used, or a 0.5% solution of sodium hypochlorite. The sterilisation of blood splashes and awkward corners and crevices is mostly done with a blow lamp.

The destruction of all products concerned with slaughter is of great importance – hoofs, horns, blood, viscera, fat and hide.

Clothing, aprons, etc. may be disinfected by steam in an autoclave at 7–kg pressure for half an hour.

Judgement: Total rejection.

Azoturia

This is a condition in horses, the cause of which is not known. The muscles of the hindquarters become hard and swollen. There may be a high temperature. Animals appear to be in pain, stiff and reluctant to move. Urine is of a wine red colour.

Judgement: This depends upon the state of the carcass.

Blackquarter or blackleg

Blackquarter is an acute infective disease of cattle and occasionally of sheep and deer, caused by *Clostridium chauvoci*. It is a soil-borne disease and is therefore more common in animals at pasture.

Susceptible animals may be infected by inoculation or more commonly by ingestion of spores. It is most common in young animals up to 2 years old in good bodily condition, and is invariably fatal.

In the ox the typical lesion is a swelling that crepitates on pressure. It develops in the subcutaneous tissue and spreads rapidly.

Lesions occur most commonly in the large muscles of the fore and hindquarters, hence the name blackleg or blackquarter. However, many other muscles may be affected, e.g. tongue, masseter muscles, diaphragm and intercostal muscles.

On post-mortem examnation the connective tissue is infiltrated with a yellow gelatinous substance that is haemorrhagic and gassy. The muscle is blackish-red and oedematous at the periphery of the swelling but dry and sponge-like due to gas spaces in the centre. There is a strong smell like rancid butter or cheese. The lymph nodes are enlarged and haemorrhagic.

Judgement: Total rejection.

Botriomycosis

This is a term used to describe chronic abscess formation in the horse caused by *Staphylococcus aureus*. The abscesses most commonly occur in the spermatic cord after castration and in the shoulder region in heavy horses owing to ill fitting collars.

Judgement: Local trimming.

Bovine spongiform encephalopathy (BSE)

BSE was formally diagnosed in cattle in the United Kingdom in 1986. Spongiform encephalopathies amongst other animals were well known, e.g. scrapie in sheep was first recognised over 250 years ago. In cattle it was recognised as possibly a new disease. It then became an epidemic amongst cattle herds in the UK. The epidemic peaked in early 1993 when over 1000 suspected cases per week were being reported. With the introduction of controls the number of suspected cases in January 1997 dropped to less than 150 cases per week. Scientists believe that the BSE epidemic will have faded close to extinction by 2001.

The disease is fatal to cattle and the symptoms are hypersensitivity, nervousness, aggressiveness, e.g. vigorous kicking if handled, and death. During ante-mortem inspection it is stressed that suspected cases should not be handled or approached because of the unpredictable and possibly dangerous behaviour of affected animals.

A number of theories have been developed about the cause of BSE. The current theory is that BSE is caused by a prion (rogue protein), and that it originally infected cattle via animal feed. The animal feed contained mammalian meat and bone material (MBM), particularly MBM containing scrapie-infected sheep carcasses. MBM was used as a source of protein and was commercially rendered from abattoir and knacker's yard waste. Changes to the rendering process in the early 1980s are thought to have been the cause. Other species including zoo animals, e.g. antelopes, are also believed to have contracted the disease in the same way. The feed ban prohibited the feeding of feedstuffs containing MBM to ruminants.

The concern now is that BSE can cause the human form of spongiform encephalopathy, Creutzfeldt Jakob Disease (CJD). This concern was prompted by reports in *The Lancet* during 1996 of a new variant of CJD. Since May 1990 all CJD cases have been investigated by a surveillance unit. Ten cases of those investigated were found to have a profile different from that which would normally be expected for CJD cases due to their young age. At post-mortem a plaque was present throughout the cerebellum and cerebrum of the brains which had nev er been seen in CJD cases previously. The authors of the article in *The Lancet* concluded that the new form of CJD was consistent with BSE being a causal factor, although the number of cases was thought to be too small to prove a link.

A number of checks are carried out at slaughter, rendering, storage and disposal of animals which aim to ensure that potentially BSE-infected material cannot enter the human food chain, contaminate the environment, or otherwise affect public health and safety. The main responsibility rests with the State Veterinary Service (SVS) and the Meat Hygiene Service (MHS). However, the Environment Agency, local authorities, water companies and the Health and Safety Executive (HSE) all have a role.

Controls of animals infected with BSE

Any animal suspected of having BSE must be notified by the owner to the relevant SVS Animal Health Office. Animals believed to be suffering from BSE are slaughtered on the farm by SVS staff, taken to an incinerator where the head is removed and sent to a MAFF Veterinary Investigation Centre for confirmatory analysis. The rest of the carcass is incinerated.

The incinerators are authorised by MAFF to process BSE carcasses. The SVS carries out random audits to ensure that the carcasses are incinerated and the incinerator is operating properly.

Emissions from incinerators are authorised by Local Authority Environmental Health Departments or the Environment Agency. This requires monitoring of emissions, notification of results and reporting of any emissions that are outside the authorised limits.

Controls at slaughterhouses

All bovine animals are ante-mortem inspected by the MHS to check for signs of BSE. The SVS also audits these checks. There are four areas of control at the slaughterhouse:

(1)   The presentation of the animal for slaughter
(2)   The slaughter and dressing of the animal
(3)   The handling of Specified Bovine Material (SBM)
(4)   The SBM controls.

At presentation: The age is determined by checking for a maximum of two permanent incisors, or by checking the documents showing that the animal is under 30 months of age, or that it is included in the Beef Assurance scheme. The Beef Assurance scheme is a registration scheme which specialist beef producing farmers can join if they can show that their herd has never had a case of BSE and has never been exposed to the risk of BSE. It allows cattle under the scheme to be sold for slaughter for human consumption up to 42 months of age.

The identity of the animal is confirmed by checking documents and ear tags. This is normally checked in the lairage. Only MAFF-approved ear tags can be used. The kill date of the animal is recorded. Trading Standards Officers investigate any dubious documents. If there is a doubt about the age of the animal the carcass is detained with the ears. A post-mortem dentition check is also carried out by the MHS inspector.

At slaughter and dressing: During these processes the main philosophy is to remove and control contamination from SBM. Under the regulations bovine skulls, brain, spinal cord, eyes, tonsils, thymus, intestines and spleen of cattle over 6 months of age and the thymus and intestines of calves under 6 months of age are included in the definition of SBM. Therefore any brain tissue lost during slaughter is collected and disposed of as SBM. The pith rod and captive bolts are cleaned or wiped between carcasses. Any towels used to clean or wipe are also treated as SBM.

It is recommended that the tongue be removed before the head. If this is not done, then the tongue must be removed without delay after head removal. There should be no SBM contamination during tongue removal. Calf heads less than six months of age are not classed as SBM. The head should be removed without any contamination by SBM. A full head inspection is then undertaken and removed as SBM without delay. It is stained and removed from the premises.

After evisceration the carcass is inspected to ensure no rectum or spleen is left on the carcass. When the carcass is split, there should be as little bone dust produced as possible. The saw water is ducted away from the carcass to a trapped drain which collects all the small bone particles. This material is collected and disposed of as SBM. The saw is sterilised between each carcass.

The spinal cord is removed, weighed and stained. It is recommended that the corda equina is also removed even though it is not SBM. The meninges should also be removed. The vertebral canal should be inspected to ensure it is clear of spinal cord. All tools and knives used in this operation are washed and sterilised between carcasses. All material collected is placed in the SBM bin for disposal. The bovine vertebrae cannot be used as a source of mechanically recovered meat (MRM). The thymus is removed. On the neck the thymus and associated fat are removed by trimming. Thorough checks are made between the muscle bunches to ensure that all the thymus has been removed. The thymus around the heart must also be removed.

There can be up to 8 kg of SBM trim removed from each carcass. The MHS inspector thoroughly checks the carcass and weighs the SBM trim. It is an offence to present a carcass with any SBM still attached. After the final inspection the bone dust is washed off using a low pressure downward spray. The green offals and spleen are inspected in the gut room. The intestines are removed from the stomach. The spleen is removed by pulling. Any fat harvested must be double checked for SBM.

Handling the SBM: All SBM is to be stained with 0.5% dilution of patent blue 5 dye. Designated SBM tools are used to turn over the SBM whilst staining to ensure the whole surface is stained. Designated knives are to be used for SBM trimming. The use of squeegees is recommended for collecting SBM from floors.

Any bins and tools used for SBM are to be clearly marked. All fluids must be contained within the bins. Any leaking containers must be repaired. All bins and containers are to be kept clean, and stored in designated areas with a trapped drain, and the area must be regularly disinfected.

SBM controls: Thorough records are to be maintained and include: the weight of the SBM, the spinal cord weight, the number of heads, the number of sets of offal, spleens, thymus and associated fat and other fat trimmings. The records can be by weight or an accurate volume. These records are checked at the renderer and compared with the slaughterhouse records to ensure complete disposal of all SBM.

Also at slaughterhouses the over-30-month-scheme cattle are slaughtered, but separated from other animals. The SBM is removed as in other cattle and stained with the patent blue dye. The remaining carcass is stained yellow and is not used as material for human consumption. The whole carcass is destroyed.

The water companies set consent conditions covering all discharges of trade effluent to sewage treatment works. The Evironment Agency sets consent conditions for discharges into water such as rivers. The water companies and the Environment Agency monitor discharges and those which do not comply with the consent are unlawful and may be subject to prosecution.

Controls on rendering

Rendering plants are authorised by the Agriculture Department to process SBM and over-30-month carcasses. The SVS makes unannounced visits to check that all the SBM and material from 30-month animals are kept separate and are incinerated.

Controls on discharges to sewers, water and the air are those applied to slaughterhouses.

Controls on transport

MHS inspectors seal the lorries carrying SBM and over-30-month material before they leave the slaughterhouse. The transportation of MBM and tallow from SBM and over-30-month cattle is controlled by registration of the carriers by the Environment Agency. The legal duty of care applies to this controlled waste so that only authorised waste carriers can be used.

Controls on storage

The storage of carcasses prior to rendering is the responsibility of the Intervention Board Executive Agency. Storage of waste MBM and tallow from over-30-month cattle pending its disposal is controlled by a waste management licence issued by the Environment Agency.

Controls on ruminant feed

The SVS carries out random sampling of feed mills and farms to ensure the feed ban is followed.

In addition to all these controls on bovine animals the heads of sheep and goats are now treated as SBM following precautionary advice from the Spongiform Encephalopathy Advisory Committee (SEAC) in 1996. The Heads of Sheep and Goats Order 1996 prohibits the sale of sheep and goat heads (excluding the tongue) for human consumption.

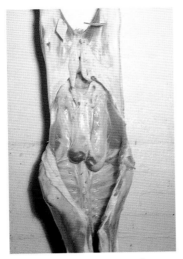

(a) Oedematous carcass of sheep

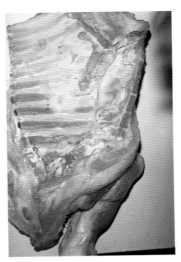

(b) Septic pleurisy in calf

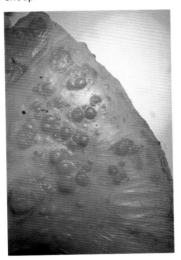

(c) Actinobacillosis of bovine tongue

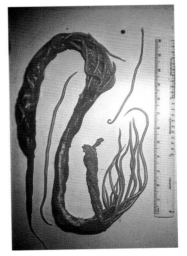

(d) *Ascaris suum* in pig intestine

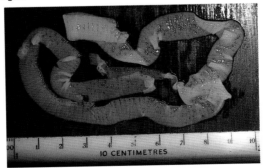

(e) *Moniezia expansa* from sheep intestine

Plate 1

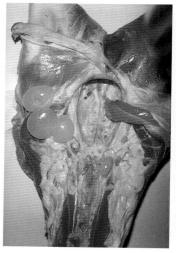

(a) Tenuicollis cysts in ewe abdomen

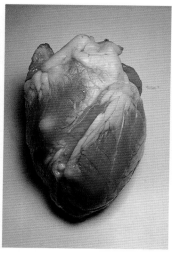

(b) *Cysticercus ovis* infection of sheep heart

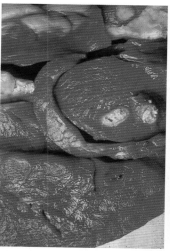

(c) *Cysticercus bovis* infection of bovine heart

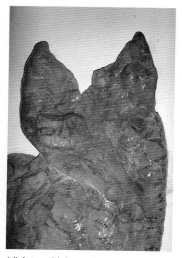

(d) Interstitial emphysema in bovine lung

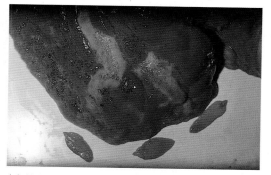

(e) *Fasciola hepatica* infection of sheep liver

Plate 2

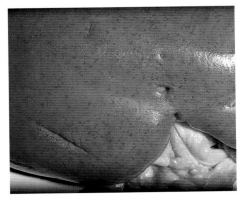

(a) Petechiae in pig kidney

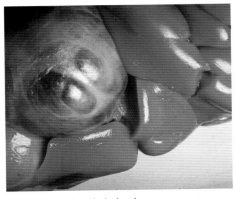

(b) Hydronephrosis in bovine kidney

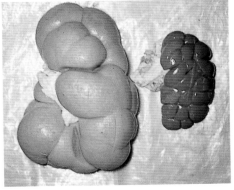

(c) Chronic nephritis in bovine kidney

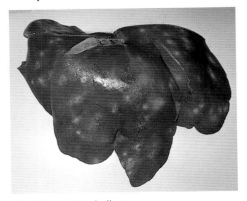

(d) Milk spot in pig liver

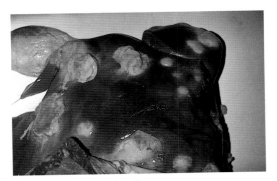

(e) Abscesses in bovine liver

Plate 3

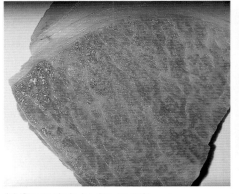

(a) Steatosis in bovine muscle

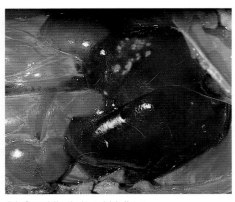

(b) Coccidiosis in rabbit liver

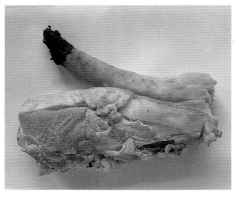

(c) 'Tail bite' and abscesses in pig

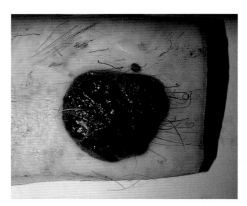

(d) Melanoma in pig skin

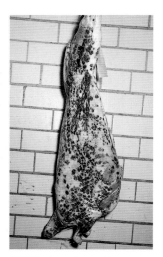

(e) Black spot mould
infection of sheep

Plate 4

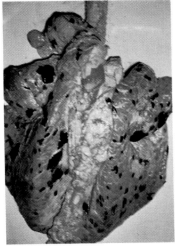

(a) Melanosis in bovine lung

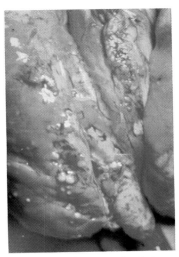

(b) Pyaemic abscesses in pig lungs

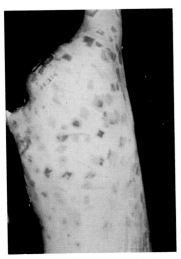

(c) 'Diamonds' in swine erysipelas

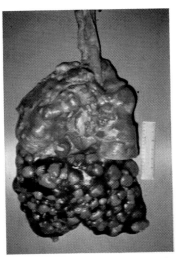

(d) Echinococcus cysts in sheep liver and lungs

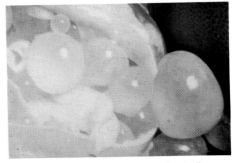

(e) Echinococcus daughter cysts in pig liver

Plate 5

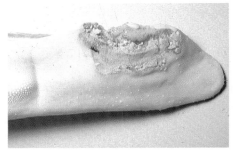

(a) Calf diptheria in tongue

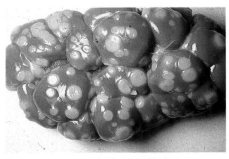

(b) Fibroplastic nephritis in calf kidney

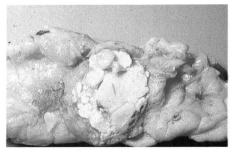

(c) Fat necrosis - bovine

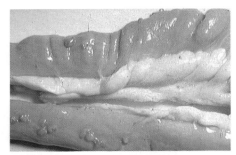

(d) 'Pimply gut' in bovine intestine

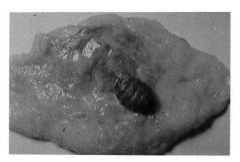

(e) Warble larva - 'licked back' - bovine

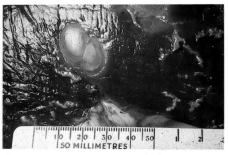

(f) Tenuicollis cysts and tracks in sheep liver

Plate 6

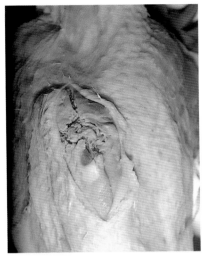

(a) Breast blister abscess

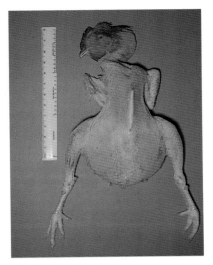

(b) *Ascites* infection

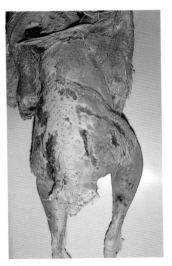

(c) Freezer burn in turkey

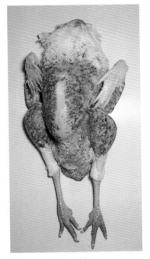

(d) Black mould infection in turkey

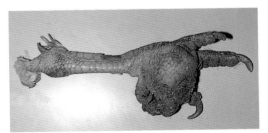

(e) Bumblefoot in turkey

Plate 7

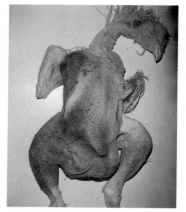

(a) Bruising in fowl

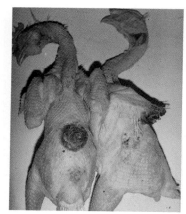

(b) Cannibalism in fowl

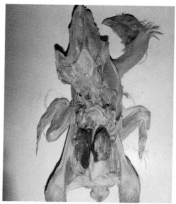

(c) *E. coli* septicaemia in fowl

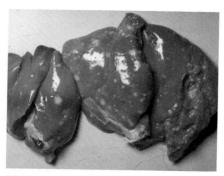

(d) Lymphoid leukosis livers in fowl

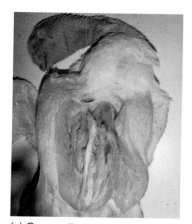

(e) Oregon disease in turkey

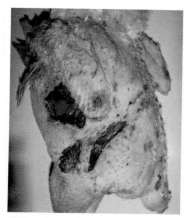

(f) Tread wounds in turkey

Plate 8

Bovine virus diarrhoea (BVD)

This is caused by a virus. Initial infection of calves and older cattle may cause diarrhoea, nasal discharge, ulcers in the mouth and salivation. Abortion is common. Infection with a second strain of the virus can cause mucosal disease.

Judgement: Total rejection.

Brucellosis

Brucellosis is the collective name for a group of diseases caused by the *Brucella* species of bacteria. *Br. abortus* causes contagious abortion in cattle. *Br. suis* causes abortion in pigs and *Br. melitensis* causes abortion in goats.

Bovine brucellosis or contagious abortion in cattle is spread mainly by contaminated uterine discharges. *Brucella abortus* can settle in the udder and be excreted in the milk, but it causes no visible lesions in the mammary tissue. In the pregnant uterus, which is the predilection site, the cotyledons are necrotic, soft, yellow grey in colour and covered by a brown exudate. The fetus is usually aborted during the 7th or 8th month of pregnancy. The fetus may be oedematous with blood-tinged subcutaneous fluid.

Br. abortus on post-mortem inspection is characterised by clumps of pus between the uterine membrane and fetal membrane. The maternal and fetal cotyledons are covered with a grey or yellow purulent material. The bovine testicle may also be affected.

Brucellosis testing is done on the farm. If a positive test result is given, the animal is sent for slaughter. This forms part of the eradication programme.

As brucellosis can be contracted by humns (undulant fever) from brucella-positive cattle, care should be taken during slaughter so that the uterus is not opened and that the udder is removed intact so that spillage of milk does not occur. Veterinary surgeons and butchers are most commonly affected.

Undulant fever may be contracted by humans drinking untreated milk or eating food made from untreated milk. Malta fever is the similar disease in humans caused by *Br. melitensis* from goat's milk.

Judgement: Reject genital organs and mammary glands.

Calf diphtheria

Calf diphtheria is a disease of young calves and is caused by *Bacteroides necrophorus*. The disease occurs by ingestion and is characterised by evil-smelling diphtheritic patches, and ulcers in the mouth, tongue, gums and pharynx. Infection may extend to the intestines to cause the typical lesions, but more commonly it causes septic broncho-pneumonia [Plate 6(a)].

Judgement: Total rejection.

Caprine arthritis encephalitis

This is a disease of goats caused by a virus. The disease is characterised by arthritis (especially of the carpal joints, hocks and stifles), encephalitis with blindness, mastitis and pneumonia.

Judgement: Total rejection.

Caseous lymphadenitis

Caseous lymphadenitis is a disease of sheep and goats caused by *Corynebacterium ovis*. It occurs mainly in Australia, New Zealand and South America and is threefore most often found in frozen imported lamb carcasses. It probably occurs occasionally in this country, as lesions indistinguishable from caseous lymphadenitis are found in home-killed sheep. The infection is probably by inoculation, as the typical lesions, in the majority of cases, are confined to the externally placed carcass lymph nodes, i.e. prescapular, precrural, superficial inguinal or supramammary and popliteal nodes.

Affected lymph nodes are generally enlarged and contain a greenish yellow gelatinous pus. Later this dries and becomes paler. In older lesions the pus becomes laminated like the layers of an onion.

Where caseous lymphadenitis is suspected, special examination is required under the Fresh Meat (Hygiene and Inspection) Regulations 1995, Schedule 10.

Judgement: Total rejection if generalised; if not, reject affected parts.

Enteritis

This is inflammation of the stomach and intestinal tract characterised by diarrhoea. It can be an acute or chronic infection.

Acute type

Often the contents of the stomach and intestines will be blood stained. The mesenteric lymph nodes are enlarged and haemorrhagic and the gall bladder is thickened. The liver may show signs of fatty degeneration and there may be blood-stained fluid in the pleural and peritoneal cavities. Petechial haemorrhages are evident in the kidneys, and the lungs are hepatised similar to septicaemia.

Judgement: Total rejection.

Chronic type

Chronic enteritis would show as discrete areas of necrosis especially around the caecum and colon; the bowel wall would be thickened with greenish yellow necrotic material. It is necessary to check for evidence of systemic infection.

Judgement: Total rejection if systemic infection, otherwise reject affected parts.

Enzootic abortion of ewes

This is caused by *Chlamydia psittaci* and accounts for about half of all the abortions in ewes. Abortion generally occurs during the last few weeks of pregnancy, resulting in dead or weak lambs. Infection is passed by the fetal membranes or by the faeces.

The main post-mortem finding is a metritis with dark red cotyledons surrounded by yellowish-grey thickened areas.

Humans can be infected by the organism and those most susceptible are shepherds, veterinary surgeons and butchers. Pregnant women are particularly at risk and should not come into contact with lambing ewes.

Judgement: Total rejection.

Enzootic bovine leukosis

Enzootic bovine leukosis is a transmissible virus disease of cattle causing leukaemia and multiple tumours (lymphosarcomas) mainly in the lymph nodes. In the live animal the disease is characterised by chronic ill health, anaemia, anorexia and weakness. Subcutaneous lymph nodes may be enlarged and palpable, generally in animals of between 4 and 8 years of age.

The disease is notifiable. The virus also affects sheep and goats but the disease is not notifiable in these animals.

Judgement: Carcasses and offal are rejected.

Enzootic pneumonia (so-called virus pneumonia)

Enzootic pneumonia is a disease of pigs caused by *Mycoplasma hyopneumoniae*.

In the vast majority of cases the lesions are confined to the ventral portions (i.e. the edges) of the lungs, particularly in the cardiac and apical lobes. The diaphragmatic lobes are far less frequently affected. The lesions are usually plum coloured. Sometimes they are greyish and have the appearance of lymphoid tissue. The pneumonic areas are clearly demarcated from the normal lung tissue and are level with or below it. Frequently pleurisy and pericarditis are present and the bronchial and mediastinal lymph nodes are enlarged and oedematous.

Judgement: Reject affected parts.

Foot and mouth disease

Foot and mouth disease is the most contagious of all animal diseases. It is caused by a filtrable virus of which there are various types. The seven major types are A, O, C, SAT 1, SAT 2, SAT 3 and Asia 1. Cattle, pigs, sheep, goats, deer and hedgehogs are susceptible to natural infection. Man is very occasionally infected and in 1966 one such case occurred in Northumberland. The disease is not endemic in Great Britain. It is introduced into the country mainly in imported frozen meat and possibly as a windborne infection across the Channel from the continent of Europe. Birds may also be implicated. Foot and mouth disease is a notifiable disease and in Britain a slaughter policy is carried out.

In the 1967–68 epidemic, caused by the O1 virus, 433 987 animals including 211 825 cattle, 113 766 pigs, 108 345 sheep and 51 goats were slaughtered. The cost in compensation was over £26 500 000.

In 1981 an outbreak was confirmed in the Isle of Wight on one farm in a herd of 166 cattle. All were slaughtered, as were 40 cattle and 200 pigs on two other farms. Sixteen other cattle from a neighbouring farm were sent to a market in Devon. All the animals were traced and slaughtered. The virus involved was type O.

Compensation paid was over £90 000. Another £50 000 was spent in clean-up operations, destruction, etc.

Symptoms
The incubation period is approximately 3–8 days. In cattle the first noticeable symptoms are dullness and depressed appetite with a rise in temperature. As the lesions develop in the mouth and on the feet, there is an increase in the secretion of saliva, which may hang from the mouth in strings, and a sudden onset of lameness. There is a disinclination for the animals to move. Cattle frequently shake their feet as if trying to remove something.

Salivation is often accompanied by a smacking or sucking sound which is characteristic. Salivation may occur in pigs and sheep but is not so noticeable.

The lesions of the disease are vesicles or blisters that, in the mouth, appear on the tongue, cheeks, gums and dental pad. In pigs the snout is often the site of lesions. The foot lesions are generally found at the junction of the skin with the hoof and between the clays. They are commonly found on the teats and skin of the udder in females. Less commonly they may be seen on the muzzle, in the nostrils, inside the vagina and on the skin of the body of pigs.

The vesicles vary in size from a pin head to half a walnut. They rupture easily and a clear fluid flows out. The mucous membrane over the vesicles looks ragged and is blanched. When the vesicles rupture they leave red-raw shallow ulcers with ragged edges. The ulcers later become yellow. The foot lesions are similar to those in the mouth except that the covering is denser. Vesicles tend to coalesce with consequent under-running of the mucous membranes. In the latter stages of the disease the clays may be shed.

Very young calves may die from enteritis without showing any other evidence.

In sheep, acute lameness of sudden onset, usually of all four feet, is characteristic. There is reluctance to rise and the sheep may adopt a crouching position. The typical lesions are found around the coronets and in the inter-digital clefts. Lesions only occasionally occur in the mouth, on the lips and dental pad.

In deer the lesions are similar to those in sheep but are generally not so severe.

In pigs the lesions and symptoms are similar to those in sheep. Thimbling of the horn of the feet, as new horn grows down the feet, occurs. Occasionally lesions occur on the tongue and snout.

The clinical disease in pigs is indistinguishable from swine vesicular disease.

If foot and mouth disease is suspected in an abattoir, it is imperative that the Divisional Veterinary Officer of the Ministry of Agriculture, Fisheries and Food be notified immediately. There should be no movement in or out of the abattoir until permission is given.

Judgement: Total rejection.

Glanders or farcy

This is a disease of horse, ass, mule and occasionally humans. It has also been encountered in carnivorous animals in zoos fed on infected horse meat. The disease is contagious and is caused by *Bacillus mallei*. The disease is usually chronic. The organism does not multiply in the bloodstream but is carried by the blood to certain predilection sites, the lung capillaries, the nasal mucous membrane or the lymph nodes. Infection occurs by ingestion of contaminated food or water and rarely through skin abrasions.

A symptom of the disease is small grey nodules in the nostrils that rapidly become ulcerative; also the submaxillary lymph node is frequently enlarged. They cause a yellowish brown blood-tinged nasal catarrh. In chronic glanders shot-like nodules the size of a pea which are grey in colour surrounded by a red area of congestion are found in the lungs. The centres degenerate to a yellowish material which is easily visible in the lung tissue.

In farcy (the skin form of glanders) the nodules resemble knotted cords. The cutaneous nodes may suppurate and become ulcerative and discharge a purulent material. The nodes are seen on the limbs or lower part of the belly.

Glanders in humans is usually caused by inoculation. Nodules develop and the lymphatic system becomes inflamed. It can spread to the nasal membranes or lungs. The disease is notifiable.

Judgement: Total rejection.

Glässer's disease

This is a disease of young pigs 5–12 weeks of age caused by *Haemophilus suis*. It is a fibrinous meningitis, polyserositis and polyarthritis. the commonest lesions are fibrinous pleurisy, fibrinous peritonitis and arthritis with an increase of synovial fluid in the joints.

Judgement: Dependent upon the severity of the lesions, but in many cases stripping of the pleura and peritoneum is sufficient.

Jöhne's disease (paratuberculosis)

Jöhne's disease is a chronic infectious disease of cattle, sheep, farmed deer and goats, caused by *Mycobacterium johnei*.

Symptoms

In cattle, diarrhoea develops early and is foul smelling and contains gas bubbles. There is wasting of the muscles of the hindquarters, loss of condition, rough coat and submaxillary oedema, and eventually the animal becomes very emaciated. The symptoms develop from 9 months of age onwards. It is a disease of animals approaching maturity, and animals of the Channel Islands breeds are the most susceptible. In sheep and goats, diarrhoea is often absent and in sheep the wool becomes harsh and pulls out easily.

In cattle the intestinal mucous membrane becomes very thickened ('thick ropes') and corrugated. It may be three or four times its normal thickness. Although the ileum is chiefly affected, the caecum, colon and rectum may also be affected. The corrugations cannot be obliterated by stretching and may show areas of congestion. Caseation occurs in sheep and goats but not in cattle and deer. The mesenteric lymph nodes are enlarged and oedematous.

The Jöhne's carcass is typical: it is emaciated with the fat showing a dead white appearance that lacks lustre and also tends to be wet and sloppy, especially by the brisket. The muscles are very wasted although there may be a fair amount of body fat still present. The muscle pits on pressure.

NB In deer it is very difficult to differentiate between Jöhne's disease and avian tuberculosis infection. Sometimes, however, in avian TB infection, caseous lesions are obvious in lymph nodes and organs.

Judgement: Dependent upon the degree of emaciation and oedema and the setting of the carcass. It is always advisable to detain the carcass for 12–24 hours before making a judgement as very often the carcass remains wet and does not set. reject intestines.

Keratitis (infectious keratoconjunctivitis or pink eye)

This is a disease of cattle caused by *Morexella bovis* and is commonest in summer and autumn when flies are abundant. Breeds of cattle with white faces, e.g. Hereford and Hereford crosses, are most commonly affected. There is uni-or bilateral injection of the corneal vessels and oedema of the conjunctiva with copious watering of the eyes. A small opacity appears in the cornea that becomes raised and ulcerated. The opacity may spread to the whole of the cornea. Complete recovery generally occurs but occasionally blindness may result.

A similar disease occurs in sheep caused by *Mycoplasma conjunctivae*.

Judgement: Reject head.

Leptospirosis

Leptospirosis is a disease caused by various types of the bacterium *Leptospira interrogans*. It can infect all the domestic animals. In cattle *L. pomona* and *L. hardjo* are the most common cause of the disease; in sheep *L. hebdomadis, L. australis* and *L. pomona* are the most common cause; in deer *L. sejroe, L. batavia,*

L. icterohaemorrhagica and *L. ballum* are the most common cause; in pigs *L. icterohaemorrhagica, pomona* and *canicola*. Jaundice (see p. 107) and abortions are the main features of the disease in animals.

The bacterium can be transmitted to humans causing Weil's disease. Abbatoir workers can be infected by *L. canicola* from pigs, causing canicola fever.

Judgement: total rejection.

Listeriosis

The disease is caused by *Listeria monocytogenes*. It affects mainly sheep, deer and cattle, but occurs in nearly all animals. It is a cause of abortion in sheep and cattle. The main effect is an encephalitis but it may assume a septicaemic form causing small necrotic lesions in the liver, spleen and heart and in the mucosae of the digestive tract and uterus. The occurrence of the disease is often associated with the feeding of silage. The organism can be spread to humans by the consumption of the milk or milk products and meat products. Soft cheeses are most commonly implicated. Pregnant women are advised not to eat soft cheeses or pâté, or to come into contact with ewes at lambing time. Infection may cause abortion or damage to the fetus.

Judgement: Total rejection.

Lymphadenitis

This is inflammation of the lymph nodes and can be acute or chronic.

Acute type
It is characterised by swelling and oedema of the lymph nodes. These will be softer than normal and are usually congested. The congestion may vary greatly depending on the disease causing the lymphadenitis. In acute swine fever the nodes are described as strawberry lymph nodes, but in anthrax the nodes are deeply congested and almost black in colour.

Chronic type
The chronic type is characterised by an increase in fibrous connective tissue and in the size of the affected node, e.g. actinobacillosis.

Judgement: Total rejection for both types.

Maedi-Visna

Maedi-Visna is a slowly acting virus disease of sheep with a prolonged incubation period. It was first diagnosed in Finland. Symptoms are not generally seen in sheep under 3 years of age. These are a loss of condition, dyspnoea, mastitis, lameness and occasionally paralysis. It is frequently fatal.

At post-mortem the lungs are enlarged and firm and do not collapse when the thorax is opened. Very often impressions of the ribs are seen on the caudal lobes. The lungs have a yellowish grey or bluish grey tinge. The cut surface is dry and homogeneous and on palpation feels like a rubber sponge. The lymph nodes are greatly enlarged. The visceral pleura is thickened and more opaque than normal.

The udder is enlarged and indurated. There may be a non-suppurative arthritis of the carpal and tarsal joints. Occasionally the central nervous system is affected causing a progressive paralysis.

Judgement: Total rejection.

Malignant catarrhal fever

Malignant catarrhal fever is a fatal disease of cattle and farmed deer that occasionally occurs in the UK. It is caused by a virus that is carried by sheep but does not cause any symptoms in them.

There are acute inflammatory changes in the mucous membranes. The symptoms include mucopurulent discharges from the eyes and nostrils, salivation, conjunctivitis, keratitis and often blindness, enlargement of lymph nodes, sloughing of the buccal and nasal mucosae and diarrhoea.

In farmed deer the disease may be very acute, and infected animals may die within 24 hours of showing symptoms.

Judgement: Total rejection.

Mucosal disease

Mucosal disease occurs in cattle of 6 months to 2 years old that are carrying the BVD virus. It is caused by infection with a second strain of the BVD virus. It is invariably fatal. Erosions occur in the mouth, especially on the gums and tongue and on the mucous membranes of the nostrils and nasal cavities. In some cases there is desquamation of the muzzle with consequent purulent exudates. Erosions of the mucosae occur throughout the entire alimentary tract. Lesions also occur in the interdigital clefts. The animals become lame and are found lying down.

Judgement: Total rejection.

Orf (contagious pustular dermatitis or malignant aphtha)

Orf is a disease common to sheep and goats and is caused by a virus.

Outbreaks of the disease are commonest in spring and summer. Sheep of any age may be attacked but it is prevalent in lambs up to a year old.

The disease is characterised by pustular or ulcerative lesions of the skin and mucous membranes, which are often confined to the lips and surrounding tissues, but may affect almost any other part of the body, e.g. feet, skin and genitalia.

The disease is communicable to humans, and slaughtermen and meat inspectors are particularly liable to infection because of the skinning of sheep heads and the examination of sheep's tonsils.

Judgement: If generalised, the carcass and offal are rejected. Otherwise, local trimming and rejection of affected parts is sufficient.

Pulmonary adenomatosis (Jaagsiekte or driving sickness)

This is a respiratory disease of sheep aged between 5 months and 11 years. It is a virus disease and has occurred in the east of Scotland for many years.

Affected sheep show marked respiratory distress, often with a frothy muco-purulent nasal discharge. There is marked loss of weight and affected sheep usually die within a few weeks.

As the name implies, there is tumour formation in the lungs.

Judgement: Carcass and offal are rejected.

Pig paratyphoid or necrotic enteritis

Pig paratyphoid is a disease of young pigs up to 22 weeks old and is caused by *Salmonella cholerae suis.* The acute septicaemic forms are usually seen in sucking pigs up to 3 weeks old and are therefore not seen in abattoirs.

The enteric and pneumonic forms are the types most commonly seen and the lesions are as follows:

(1) Pneumonia.
(2) Skin lesions – circular areas of scab about 2 cm in diameter most commonly found on the flanks. Unlike ringworm, the centre of the lesion shows no tendency to heal and the superficial lymph nodes are enlarged.
(3) Necrotic enteritis of the large intestine is characterised by diphtheresis and necrosis.

Judgement: Carcasses and offal should be rejected as *Salmonella cholerae suis* can be the cause of a serious type of food poisoning in humans.

'Q' (query) fever

'Q' fever is caused by a rickettsia, *Coxiella burnetti.* The disease is widespread in sheep and cattle. In these animals it is often of a very mild type. In humans there is an acute fever with headache and an atypical pneumonia. Infection is usually by contaminated dust from sheep, goats and cattle. The highest risk is exposure to sheep fetal membranes. Humans have also been affected by exposure to wild rabbits.

Recently, abortion in cattle and sheep has been found to be caused by *C. burnetti.*

Judgement: Total rejection.

Rabies

Rabies is caused by a virus which possesses an affinity for nervous tissues such as the brain and spinal cord. It is a notifiable acute infective disease which is transmitted by a bite from an infected animal. Wounds to the lips, cheek and nose are especially dangerous. It is mainly a disease of carnivorous animals. It has a long incubation period of 2–6 weeks but this may be 6 months or more. Rabid cattle, sheep and goats initially show symptoms of sexual excitement, bellowing and aggressive behaviour. This leads to eventual paralysis and death. Pigs show a pronounced irritation and wander aimlessly, followed by aggression, paralysis and death.

Judgement: Total rejection.

Salmonellosis

Salmonellosis is caused by bacteria of the salmonella group of which there are over 2000 known types. They are widely distributed in animals, birds and reptiles. Their normal habitat is the intestinal tract and they are therefore excreted in the faeces. The types that commonly cause disease in animals are *S. dublin*, *S. typhimurium*, *S. enteritidis* and *S. cholerae suis*. *Salmonella dublin* has been reported as the cause of dermatitis on the arms of veterinary surgeons after the obstetrical examination of cows.

In calves the disease (mainly by *S. dublin*, 62%, and *S. typhimurium*, 34%) causes an enteritis. The characteristic symptoms are a brown or pasty diarrhoea, dullness, dehydration and loss of appetite with a high temperature. In older animals it causes fever, loss of appetite, diminution in milk yield and a severe diarrhoea that is foul smelling and may contain blood.

The meat from affected animals may contain salmonellae and so cause food poisoning in humans. As there are no characteristic post-mortem lesions this emphasises the importance of ante-mortem inspection.

The inspection and judgement, particularly of calves and pigs showing any sign of fever or systemic disturbance, should be severe.

Bacteriological examination of suspected carcasses should be a routine procedure.

Prolonged lairaging of animals should be discouraged as this tends to build up the salmonella population with consequent infection of more animals. This fact has been recognised in the Fresh Meat (Hygiene and Inspection) Regulations 1995, which limit the time in lairage of animals to 72 hours.

Salmonellosis is without doubt the most difficult problem in meat inspection. The only safe procedure would be to bacteriologically examine every carcass, but of course this is not practicable.

Judgement: Total rejection when acute infection.

Scrapie

Scrapie is a fatal disease of sheep and goats caused by a virus-like particle. The incubation period is 18 months to 5 years. Lambs and kids are probably infected by contact with or by eating fetal membranes. The disease is characterised by a slow progressive degeneration of the central nervous system.

The symptoms are an irregular gait and an intense irritation of the skin causing the animal to rub against fences, bushes and trees (hence the name scrapie). The fleece has a ragged apearance and there are often skin sores. Collapse and death eventually ensue.

Recently a new disease of cattle has appeared, bovine spongiform encephalopathy (see p. 119), which the Government and MAFF scientists believe is almost certainly due to the feeding of animal food containing protein from scrapie-infected sheep.

Judgement: Total rejection.

Strangles

This is a disease of horses caused by *Streptococcus equi*. Abscesses occur in the lymph nodes of the head, particularly in the submaxillaries. There is often a copious yellow nasal discharge. Rarely the condition spreads causing abscesses in the lungs, liver, spleen and kidneys.

Judgement: Total rejection if widespread, but mostly it is only necessary to reject the head.

Swine erysipelas

Swine erysipelas is an acute infectious disease of pigs caused by *Erysipelothrix rhusiopathiae (E. insidiosa)*. Humans may become infected by handling infected pork. In humans it is called erysipeloid.

There are three readily distinguishable forms of swine erysipelas, although these three can merge into one another:

(1)   urticarial or mild type
(2)   acute or septicaemic type
(3)   chronic type.

Urticarial type

(1)   'Diamonds' on skin – these are purple or red, slightly swollen diamond-shaped areas 1.5–5 cm across [Plate 5(c)].
(2)   A few petechial haemorrhages in the kidneys.

Acute type

(1)   Acute inflammatory areas on the skin – ears, neck, abdomen and buttocks.
(2)   Petechial haemorrhages in kidneys and maybe in lungs and intestines.
(3)   Carcass is fevered, e.g. haemorrhagic lymph nodes and the fat is red.
(4)   Spleen is enlarged.

Chronic type

(1)   Arthritis – particularly stifle joints and other joints of hind legs. On puncturing the joints a typical chocolate-brown synovial fluid escapes.
(2)   Internal iliac lymph nodes, enlarged and dark red in colour.
(3)   Verrucose endocarditis – cauliflower-like lesions on the heart valves. Similar lesions may be caused by streptococci. The left side of the heart is more often affected than the right side.
(4)   Verrucae in kidneys – these are typical large greyish infarcts in the kidneys.
(5)   Typical venous congestion of lungs: lungs have a marble-like appearance owing to obvious interlobular septae.

Occasionally the chronic type breaks down into the acute type again.
Judgement: In mild type – remove affected parts, i.e. skin and possibly kidneys.
In acute type – total rejection.
In chronic type – judgement depends on how widespread, but very often only affected organs and arthritic portions rejected.

Swine fever

Swine fever is a notifiable disease. A slaughter policy is in operation.
The disease is caused by a virus. It is an acute, highly infective disease and the typical lesions are petechial haemorrhages. There are two types, (1) acute and (2) hronic.
Outbreaks are usually attributed to the feeding of unprocessed waste food containing imported pig-meat products.

Acute type
Petechial haemorrhages are widespread and occur in kidneys, intestines, lungs, liver, larynx, skin, pleura and peritoneum. The haemorrhages in the kidneys even extend to the pelvis of the kidney, and the skin petechiae show in the form of a rash that may be almost black in colour. The lymph nodes are severely congested and are almost black in colour. The carcass is fevered.

Chronic type
The only lesion in the chronic type may be the so-called 'button ulcer' in the intestine. The common site for button ulcers is in the region of the ileo-caecal

valve but they may be found anywhere in the large intestine and occasionally in the small intestine. Necrotic skin lesions are occasionally present.

When swine fever is found in an abattoir, it is important that the Divisional Veterinary Officer to the Ministry of Agriculture, Fisheries and Food be notified immediately so that appropriate measures can be taken to deal with the situation.

Judgement: Total rejection for both types.

Swine vesicular disease

Swine vesicular disease is a notifiable disease of pigs caused by a virus. The lesions are similar to those of foot and mouth disease, i.e. vesicles up to 2 cm in diameter that appear on the feet, lips, snout and tongue. There is an initial rise in temperature and the pigs appear to be ill. The foot lesions cause lameness.

The first outbreak of the disease in England occurred in December 1972 and at first was mistakenly diagnosed as foot and mouth disease from which it is clinically indistinguishable. However, the virus of swine vesicular disease only affects pigs whereas the foot and mouth disease virus affects pigs, cattle, deer, sheep and goats.

The disease is notifiable, and a slaughter policy is carried out.

Judgement: Total rejection.

Tetanus

Tatanus is an infective disease caused by the anerobic, soil-borne bacillus, *Clostridium tetani.* There are no diagnostic post-mortem lesions and therefore it is a disease in which ante-mortem inspection is of the greatest value. All animals including humans can be infected. It is commonest, however, in horses, sheep and pigs. Infection is by inoculation and so is associated with wounds especially of the deep penetrating type, e.g. 'picked up nail' wounds in horses' feet. The depth of such a wound is ideal for the multiplication of the anaerobic bacilli. The neurotoxin produced by the bacilli causes the typical muscular spasms. When the masseter muscles are affected, the jaws are locked and the animal is unable to swallow, hence the name 'lockjaw'.

Docking and castration wounds are other means of entry into the tissues by the bacilli, and so lambs and piglets are fairly commonly affected. Animals that are infected generally bleed badly when slaughtered.

All personnel working in slaughterhouses should be vaccinated against tetanus.

Judgement: Total rejection.

Tuberculosis

Tuberculosis is a chronic infectious disease of humans and animals caused by *Mycobacterium tuberculosis.* There are three common types of the tubercle bacillus:

(1)   The human type – *M. tuberculosis*
(2)   The bovine type – *M. bovis*
(3)   The avian type – *M. avium*.

There is a fourth type that affects fish.

(1)   Human type. This affects humans, but can also affect cattle and pigs to a much lesser extent. It only importance in animals is that it causes reaction to the tuberculin test in cattle.
(2)   Bovine type. This affects humans, cattle, deer and pigs. It is much the most virulent type for cattle and pigs.

   Bovine tuberculosis in deer has occurred mainly in farmed animals in association with imported deer. One outbreak has occurred in a wild herd of sika deer in Dorset in an area in which there is a history of bovine tuberculosis in cattle and badgers. Another outbreak has occurred in a herd of park fallow deer in Warwickshire. The disease was found in carcasses at the annual cull. The source has not been identified.

   Outbreaks of tuberculosis among cattle in the south-west of England have occurred in six herds, and in spite of the usual tuberculin testing and slaughter policy it is proving difficult to eradicate the disease. This is the only area in Great Britain that is not free of tuberculosis in cattle. It was in 1974 that badgers in the area were found to be affected with bovine tuberculosis and were contaminating the pastures with *Mycobacterium bovis*. Over 200 badger sets were found. Gassing of badgers was instituted in an attempt to eliminate them. This policy is apparently meeting with success.
(3)   Avian type. This affects birds, pigs, deer and, to a much lesser extent, cattle. Avian tuberculosis in pigs, as well as being caused by *M. avium*, may also be caused by *M. intracellularae*, which is found in wood shavings and sawdust. Wild deer are particularly susceptible to the avian type.

   Until recently tuberculosis was the cause of by far the greatest amount of rejection of bovine and porcine meat and offal in this country. Now tuberculosis is very rarely seen in the abbatoir except in the lymph nodes of the pig's head and the mesenteric lymph nodes, when the infection is nearly always of the avian type. There have been recent reports of avian TB in pigs following the use of feed containing peat which was infected by bird droppings.

   It is interesting to note that sheep are very rarely infected with tuberculosis.

   Cases of suspected bovine tuberculosis in cattle and deer must be reported to the Animal Health Division of the Ministry of Agriculture.

   Although bovine tuberculosis in cattle and pigs is now almost a thing of the past in the UK, it is a classical type of disease and illustrates how bacteria can enter the body, spread and cause disease.

Modes of infection

The routes by which tubercle bacilli gain entrance to the body are:

(1) respiration
(2) ingestion
(3) inoculation
(4) congenital
(5) genital – infection by way of the genital organs.

(1) Respiration. This is by far the commonest route of infection in cattle. Cows, particularly in cowsheds, are infected by a cow with pulmonary tuberculosis (open type). One cow so affected can very soon infect all the others in the shed.

   When a bovine is infected by the respiratory route, primary lesions appear in the lung substance and/or lymph nodes of the lungs or lymph nodes of the head (see drainage areas of lymph nodes, pp. 31–41).

(2) Ingestion. This is the commonest route of infection in pigs and the second commonest route in cattle. Infection is taken in by the mouth, and the primary lesions can occur in tonsils, lymph nodes of the head, intestine and mesenteric lymph nodes.

(3) Inoculation. This is a relatively rare way of infection but can occur either:

   (a) when tuberculous material comes into contact with a wound
   (b) when contaminated teat instruments are used on cows.

(4) Congenital. This occurs in calves from cows with tuberculosis of the uterus.
(5) Genital. This is transmitted and acquired during copulation, either from cow to bull or bull to cow. It can also be transmitted by contaminated uterine instruments.

Pathogenesis of tuberculosis

Tubercle bacilli when they enter the body produce a primary lesion generally in the respiratory or digestive tract. Following this, lesions appear in the associated lymph nodes. The primary lesion may be difficult to find, especially in the intestine. In the lungs the lesion is generally in the substance of the lung at the termination of a bronchiole. The body tissues generally have specific reactions to different bacilli. In the case of tubercle baccilli, phagocytic cells proliferate around the multiplying bacilli resulting in the formation of a nodule or 'tubercle'. Multinucleated giant cells also appear and the lesion increases in size owing to the destruction of the normal tissue and the fusion of adjacent tubercles. The lesions are microscopic to begin with and are normally only visible to the naked eye in about 3 weeks. They have a translucent greyish appearance at first and this is best seen in miliary tuberculosis of the lung. The lesions then become necrotic and opaque or yellowish-white in appearance. Necrosis is followed by caseation in which the necrotic tissue becomes cheesy in texture. Sometimes fibrous tissue forms at the periphery of the lesion forming a capsule limiting the local spread of the disease process. Calcification may then follow.

At this stage the defences of the body may be so mobilised that no further spread takes place and the infection is localised. However, if the defences are overcome, further spread can take place by the following means:

(1) By local contact, e.g. from lung substance to visceral pleura and then to parietal pleura.
(2) By natural passages in the body, e.g. from lung to intestine, i.e. sputum is coughed up the trachea to the pharynx or mouth and swallowed.
(3) By lymphatic spread along lymph vessels to lymph nodes and then to other lymph nodes in the lymph flow.
(4) By haematogenous spread, i.e. bloodstream. This occurs when a tuberculous lesion erodes into a blood vessel or when tubercle bacilli are carried into the venous blood system by the lymph (see p. 32). If large numbers of bacilli enter the bloodstream, miliary tuberculosis results, which is characterised by millet-seed-sized lesions that appear throughout the organs of the body, especially the lungs, kidneys, liver and spleen. In miliary tuberculosis of the pig it is not uncommon to find no visible lesions in the lymph nodes of the carcass.

   If small numbers of bacilli enter the bloodstream, it is possible that lesions may be found in situations far removed from the main site. For example, it is not uncommon to find secondary lesions in the hindquarter lymph nodes, e.g. popliteal, as a result of haematogenous spread from a tuberculous lesion in the lung.

   If the animal does not die from the acute miliary type, the condition may become chronic, in which case the disease involves the pleura and peritoneum ('grapes') and various organs in which the lesions are of a caseous or calcified nature owing to the deposition of calcium. The body defences may be adequate and the disease becomes quiescent or healing takes place. However, reinfection may take place and disease flares up again or some of the lesions may break down and acute miliary tuberculosis results.

   Reinfection or breakdown can occur when the body is weakened in some way, e.g. by starvation or pregnancy.

Congenital tuberculosis in calves
This is often generalised, and lesions are found in the carcass lymph nodes, lungs, kidneys and splenic substance. Carcass and offal are rejected.

Lesions of tuberculosis in deer

(1) Bovine type. The retropharyngeal lymph nodes are most commonly affected. They may be enlarged and paler in colour than normal, and may

contain large amounts of pus. Lesions are also frequent in the lungs, and calcification is common.

(2)   Avian type. This affects mainly the mesenteric lymph nodes, the wall of the intestines, liver and the subcutaneous tissue. The mesenteric lymph nodes are enlarged and firm. The lymph vessels are thickened and tortuous with greyish-white nodules and are easily seen. Miliary nodules may be found in the liver. Tuberculous abscesses containing soft creamy pus are common.

The lesions in the subcutaneous tissue may be numerous and widely spread. They often contain pus.

Judgement: If generalised or associated with emaciation, total rejection. If localised, reject affected parts.

For judgement in cases of tuberculosis, reference should be made to the Fresh Meat (Hygiene and Inspection) Regulations 1995, Schedule 10.

Yersiniosis

Yersiniosis is an important disease of farmed deer. It occurs mostly in young animals. It is caused by *Yersinia (Pasteurella) pseudotuberculosis*. Death can be sudden but typical symptoms are a watery fetid diarrhoea and rapid loss of condition. Post-mortem lesions are haemorrhagic gastroenteritis, with oedema of the walls of the intestine. The mesenteric lymph nodes are oedematous and necrotic.

Judgement: Total rejection.

Chapter 16
Parasitic Diseases

Parasites

A parasite is an organism that lies on or in another organism, the host, derives nourishment from it and confers no advantage in return.

Parasitic worms may cause the death of the host but generally the result is more insidious, leading to respiratory and digestive disturbances and thus loss of condition.

Parasites affect the host in various ways:

(1) By blood sucking, e.g. *Haemonchus contortus*, a worm found in the abomasum of sheep, if numerous causes anaemia in the sheep.
(2) By injury to tissues, e.g. *Fasciola hepatica* (fluke) causes cirrhosis of the liver in cattle.
(3) By robbing the host of its food, e.g. *Ascaris suum* in young pigs.
(4) By producing toxins that injure the host, e.g. most intestinal parasites.

The most important parasites in meat inspection, and this applies to bacteria also, ar those that are transmissible to humans, by consumption of the flesh of affected animals or by coming into contact with such flesh. Other parasites, though not causing disease in humans, may render such flesh or organs repugnant and therefore not fit for sale, e.g. sarcocysts in muscles and 'milk spots' in pig's liver.

The parasites of importance in meat inspection are classified as follows:

(1) *Nematodes* or roundworms
(2) *Cestodes* or tapeworms
(3) *Trematodes* or flukes
(4) *Protozoa* or single-celled organisms
(5) *Arthropoda* or mites, flies, etc.

The nematodes

For convenience these are put into three groups, (1) intestinal worms, (2) lung worms, and (3) connective tissue worms.

Intestinal worms

Ascaris suum (A. lumbricoides)

This is a large worm – males 15–25 cm × 3 mm, females 41 cm × 5 mm, smooth and yellowish-white in colour – that inhabits the small intestine of the pig, in which it is very common. It has been recorded in stomach, large intestine and bile ducts.

Life cycle: The sexes are separate and the female lays large quantities of eggs – up to 200 000 per day. The eggs pass out in the faeces of the pig. They are not immediately infective and only become so when larvae develop in the egg. This can take 16–50 days according to the conditions. Infection of the pig takes place by ingestion of the larvae-containing eggs. The intestinal juices of the pig dissolve the walls of the eggs and the larvae are freed. The larvae burrow through the intestinal wall and reach the liver by way of the portal circulation. Many larvae penetrate the liver capillaries, moving thence to the hepatic vein and on via the blood circulation to lungs. Some larvae are retained in the liver and cause chronic focal interstitial hepatitis or, as it is commonly known, 'milk spot' [Plate 3(d)]. The peak incidence of 'milk spot' livers is in July and August. The larvae that are filtered out by the lung capillaries bore their way through the capillary walls into the alveoli of the lungs and are carried up the bronchi by the ciliated epithelium or by coughing. They reach the larynx and pharynx and are swallowed. In the intestines they develop in 8–9 weeks into mature male and female worms [Plate 1(d)]. The journey from intestine and back to intestine takes about 14 days.

The passage of the larvae through the liver and the lungs and the absorption of toxins can cause considerable systemic disturbances: fever, coughing, 'pot-bellied' appearance and stunted growth.

It is possible that humans may become infected by *Ascaris suum* but not by eating meat, only by swallowing infective eggs.

Ascaris suum is found rarely in sheep and in the calf.

Judgement: Usually only the 'milk spot' livers are rejected.

Parascaris equorum

Parascaris equorum is found quite commonly in the horse. The males measure 15–28 cm long and the females up to 50 cm × 8 mm.

Life cycle: Similar to *A. suis.* Infected foals may have a severe enteritis with diarrhoea with resultant debility.

Haemonchus contortus, Trichostrongylus axei and Ostertagia ostertagi

These are found in the abomasum and intestines of sheep and can cause a severe gastroenteritis. *Haemonchus contortus* is the largest of the group, being 10–30 mm long, reddish in colour and about the thickness of a pin.

Different species of *Haemonchus*, *Trychostrongylus* and *Ostertagia* occur in the abomasum and small intestine of deer but appear to be of little importance.

Life cycle: An infected sheep may pass millions of eggs per day. Under suitable conditions these develop into larvae, which become infective in 1–3 weeks. When swallowed, these pass to the abomasum where they become adult in 2–4 weeks.

Heavily infested sheep become anaemic, emaciated and oedematous, the oedema being particularly well seen under the lower jaw ('bottle jaw').

Haemonchus contortus, Trichostrongylus axei and *Ostertagia ostertagi* similarly affect cattle, particularly calves, and *Ostertagia* causes gastritis with pin-head-sized lesions in the abomasum.

Judgement: Dependent upon degree of anaemia, oedema and emaciation.

Hyostrongulus rubidus

This is a small red worm about 4–10 mm in length and very fine and threadlike. It is found in the pig's stomach and can give rise to a severe gastritis. It may best be seen at post-mortem examination of a freshly killed pig by examing carefully the mucosa of the stomach.

Judgement: Reject stomach.

Nematodirus filicollis and Nematodirus battus

Nematodirus filicollis occurs in the small intestine of deer and is common but of low pathogenicity.

Nematodirus battus is more pathogenic than *N. filicollis* but is rare in deer and generally in small numbers.

Oesophagostomum radiatum

It measures 12–21 mm × 0.45 mm. This causes 'pimply gut' in caecum and colon in cattle. The nodules vary in size from a pin head to a pea and are greyish white in colour and cause distinct elevations of the intestinal mucous membrane (Plate 6(d)].

Judgement: Reject intestines.

Oesophagostomum dentatum

It measures 8–14 mm × 0.5 mm. This affects pigs in the same way. The nodules render the intestines valueless for the preparation of sausage skins.

Judgement: Reject intestines.

Oesophagostomum columbianum

It measures 12–21 mm × 0.45 mm. This causes 'pimply gut' in sheep in tropical and sub-tropical countries, but not in Britain.

Life cycle: The eggs of the *Oesophagostomum* genus are passed in the faeces and hatch to give rise to a first-stage larva.

A further developmental phase takes place and under optimum conditions the infective third larval stage is reached in about a week. Infection takes place by ingestion of the larvae, which cast their sheaths in the intestine before they penetrate into the wall and form the characteristic nodules within which the third and fourth larval stages complete their development. Finally, the young adult worm regains the lumen of the large intestine where it develops to maturity.

Trichinella spiralis

This is a small worm 1.5–4 mm long, which in the adult form lives in the intestines of mammals and the larval form in the muscular tissue, when it causes, in humans particularly, a serious disease called trichinoisis or trichiniasis.

The adult worm is foun in the intestine of pig, rat, humans and other mammals. The rat is the animal most commonly affected in this country. Pigs become infected by eating affected rats or swill containing infected pork, and humans become infected by eating raw or improperly cooked pork or pork products. In humans the disease is commonest in Germany because so much raw or partly cooked or smoked sausage is eaten in that country. Many people in the Arctic, especially in Greenland, are infected by eating the flesh of infected polar bears, walruses, seals, etc.

In 1981, 46 cases, including one death, were diagnosed in New York. All the cases were associated with eating ethnic dishes that contained raw or partially cooked pork. Some of the cases were associated with eating home-made pork sausage.

In 1982, trichinosis was diagnosed in wild boars, various rat species, voles, polecats, pine martens, weasels and hedgehogs in Belgium. Live trichinellae were found in the carcass of a musk rat that had been frozen at –34°C for 35 days.

Life cycle: Adult worms are only found in the small intestines of animals that have recently eaten infected meat, i.e. muscle containing larvae. The gastric juice dissolves the cyst walls and the larvae are liberated. They develop into sexually mature adults in the intestine. The males soon die and in 14 days the majority of worms left are females. These live for about 2 months, penetrate the intestine and each gives birth to about 1500 larvae in the lymph spaces. The larvae enter the lymph stream and from thence move to the bloodstream. They are then spread widely by the arterial blood vessels throughout the muscles of the body. The larvae have a predilection for striped muscles. They enter the muscle fibres and enlarge in size and then curl up within the muscle fibres into the typical spiral form. It is from this spiral formation that the worm gets its name. Tissue reaction follows, and the larvae become enclosed in oval muscle cysts with their long axis parallel to the muscle fibres. They measure about 0.5×0.25 mm. The cysts tend to become calcified but can remain alive for many years. The life cycle is completed when the infected muscle is eaten by another animal.

The cysts are found in striped muscle. Those most frequently found to be affected are the diaphragm, the tongue, muscles of the larynx, and the abdominal and intercostal muscles.

Fortunately, trichinosis is rare in the UK but a severe outbreak occurred in Wolverhampton during the war (1940) in which over 500 people became infected and several died. The source was thought to be imported Chinese pork.

Unless the cysts have become calcified, they are not visible to the naked eye and it is therefore necessary to use a microscope or a trichinoscope (projection lantern). This is seldom done in the UK (except for EU export) but certain countries go to great lengths, e.g. Germany, where it is compulsory that all slaughtered pigs should be so examined. In Denmark, sows, boars and all pigs over 100 kg deadweight are examined.

The method of examination is to take out-grain-sized portions of muscle from diaphragm, tongue and pharyngeal muscles, compress them between two glass slides (called a compressorium) and examine under a magnification of 15–40 in the trichinoscope.

As this method is not by any means foolproof and very few cases are found, it seems rather unnecessary to go to the lengths that they do in Germany.

Proper cooking kills all the cysts.

Judgement: Total rejection.

Lung worms

The lung worms of cattle, sheep, pigs and horses are important in meat inspection because of the lesions they cause in the lungs.

They are all small, thread-like worms, yellowish-white in colour, and 3–5 cm long. They are found in the air passages and substance of the lungs. Their life cycles are very similar except that the *metastrongyles* and *Muellerius capillaris* require an intermediate host.

Life cycle: The eggs are laid by the adult females in the air passages and are coughed up, swallowed and passed out in the faeces. Infective larvae are swallowed by the host, after in some cases having passed through an intermediate host. The larvae penetrate the intestinal wall and then pass via the lymph and blood vessels to the lungs. There they are arrested in the capillaries and pass through into the air passages where they develop into the adult worms.

Dictyocaulus viviparus
Affects mainly calves, young cattle and deer. The worms cause bronchitis and pneumonia and are found in the bronchioles, often in very large numbers. This parasitic bronchitis is called 'husk' or 'hoose', and is a very serious condition that is often fatal.

It is much more common in farmed than wild deer.

Judgement: The lungs are rejected.

Dictyocaulus filaria
Causes a severe pneumonia in young lambs. At post-mortem the lungs show areas of pneumonia and emphysema.

Judgement: The lungs are rejected.

Dictyocaulus arnfieldi
Occurs in the bronchi of horses but generally the effects are slight.

Judgement: Reject affected parts.

Muellerius capillaris
Occurs, very often in large numbers, in the lungs of older sheep. It is also found in the lungs of deer. Snails and slugs act as intermediate hosts. It causes yellow or reddish brown, shot-like nodules and greenish grey patches in the lung substance. On palpation of the lungs the nodules feel like lead shot. Sometimes the nodules calcify. Pathogenic effects vary from slight to severe.
　　Judgement: The lungs are rejected.

Protostrongylus rufescens
Occurs occasionally in the lungs of sheep. The intermediate host is a snail. Roe deer are commonly infected. Yellowish nodules appear in the lung substance with no evidence of inflammation. The disease causes the deer to 'bark' and can cause serious losses.
　　Judgement: The lungs are rejected.

Metastrongylus apri
This is the commonest lung worm of the pig. The intermediate host is the earthworm. In young pigs it causes a severe pneumonia. Typical raised mother-of-pearl plaques are found on the lung surface.
　　Judgement: The lungs are rejected.

Metastrongylus pudendotectus and *Metastrongylus salmi*
Occur in the lungs of pigs but are not very common.
　　Judgement: In both cases the lungs are rejected.

Elaphostrongylus cervi
A protostrongyle that occurs in the lungs of deer. Nodules are scattered throughout the lung substance. It is very common in wild deer but not as common in farmed deer.
　　Judgement: The lungs are rejected.

Connective tissue worms

Onchocerca gibsoni
This work does not occur in the UK but is found in cattle in Australia, New Zealand and America. The male is 30–35 mm long and the female is 140–500 mm.
　　Onchocerciasis affects connective tissue and the typical nodules are found in the region of the brisket or stifle. The intermediate host is the midge *Culicoides pungens*.
　　In the brisket the lesions are found in the ligaments at the junction of the ribs and the costal cartilages. In the stifle region they are found in the connective tissue and tendons on the outer aspect of the joint. The nodules consist of an outer fibrous wall with a soft spongy centre up to 5 cm in diameter. The worms are very much entangled in the spongy network and it is impossible to remove an

entire female worm. In Australian meat inspection the stifle joint is opened and examined.

The infection cannot be transmitted to humans.

Judgement: Affected parts are rejected.

Onchocerca gutturosa

This is found in the UK in the connective tissue around the ligamentum nuchae or between the spleen and the rumen. The intermediate host is the biting fly *Simulium ornatum*. It is of no importance in meat inspection.

Stephanurus dentatus (the kidney worm of swine)

This roundworm occurs in tropical and sub-tropical countries. It is only found in Britain in imported pigs' kidneys.

Life cycle: Eggs are laid by the adult females in the pelvis of the kidney, in the ureters, or in cysts that are in communication with the ureters. The eggs pass out in the urine and become infective larvae on the soil. These enter the pig by ingestion or by penetrating through the skin. The larvae, by various routes, travel to the liver, bore through the capsule into the abdominal cavity and eventually penetrate the ureters. The wandering nature of the larvae can cause extensive lesions in the lymph nodes, liver, lungs, spleen, etc. These lesions are often abscesses containing greenish pus, which may also contain larvae or even adult worms.

Judgement: Dependent upon the degree of infection.

The cestodes (tapeworms)

These are parasitic worms with an elongated flat body (hence the name tapeworm) without an alimentary canal. They absorb their nourishment through their integument from the partly digested food of the host. The head or scolex is usually provided with suckers and hooks and is connected to the body by the neck in most cases. The body consists of a number of segments or proglottides, each of which contains both male and female genital organs. Eggs are formed in the segments and when these are 'ripe' they drop off from the body and are voided in the faeces.

Tapeworm eggs require an intermediate host to complete their life cycle. If tapeworms are numerous in the intestine, they may have a debilitating effect on the host but this is not generally severe. The importance of tapeworms is that their eggs may give rise to cysts in suitable hosts, causing severe damage.

Tapeworms of importance with regard to meat inspection are listed in Table 16.1.

Moniezia expansa (Fig. 16.1)

This occurs in the small intestine of sheep and occasionally cattle and goats [Plate 1(e)]. It causes scouring in lambs. It has a small head with four suckers and may

Table 16.1 Tapeworms of importance in meat inspection.

Worm	Host	Intermediate stage	Intermediate hosts	Site of larval stage
Taenia hydatigena	Dog	*Cysticercus tenuicollis*	Sheep, goat, cattle, deer and pigs	Abdominal cavity, free or attached to viscera
Echinococcus granulosus	Dog	Hydatid cyst (*Echinococcus*)	All domestic animals and man	Most parts of body especially liver and lungs
T. ovis	Dog	*Cysticercus ovis*	Sheep and goats	Heart and other muscles and lungs
Multiceps multiceps	Dog	*Coenurus cerebralis*	Sheep, goats and cattle	Central nervous system
T. pisiformis	Dog	*Cysticercus pisiformis*	Rabbits and hares	Liver, mesentery or abdominal cavity
M. serialis	Dog	*Coenurus serialis*	Rabbits and hares	Muscle tissue
T. saginata	Human	*Cysticercus bovis*	Cattle	Masseter muscles, heart, tongue, etc.
T. solium	Human	*Cysticercus cellulosae*	Pigs	Muscle tissue
Diphyllobothrium latum	Human	Plerocercoid	Fish	Muscle and other organs

attain a length of 6 m. The segments measure 1.6 cm across and are broader than long; each contains two sets of genital organs.

Life cycle: The 'ripe' segments are voided in the faeces. The eggs or ova escape from the segments, are eaten by mites of the genus *Galumna*, which live in grass. The intermediate stage of the tapeworm, the cysticercoid, develops within the mites. The life cycle is completed when cattle swallow mites containing cysticercoids.

Moniezia benedeni affects ruminants, mainly cattle. It is similar to *M. expansa* but is broader (up to 2.6 cm).

Anaplocephala species

Anaplocephala magna, A. mammiliana, and *A. perfoliata* are the tapeworms of the horse. The life cycles are similar to *M. expansa. Anaplocephala perfoliata* is

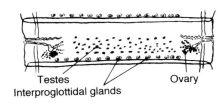

Testes   Ovary
Interproglottidal glands

Fig. 16.1 *Moniezia expansa.*

the commonest and the most important. Infection by large numbers may cause intussusception (telescoping of part of the intestine into the lumen of the adjacent part), caecal obstruction and death.

Tapeworms of the dog

These are *Echinococcus granulosus*, *Taenia hydatigena*, *T. ovis*, *T. pisiformis*. *Multiceps multiceps* and *M. serialis*. They are very important in meat inspection because their intermediate stages or cysts commonly occur in food animals.

    NB It is important to remember that all six of the dog tapeworms can be found in related wild species, e.g. the fox.

Echinococcus granulosus (Fig. 16.2)

This is the smallest tapeworm as far as we are concerned, being only about 6 mm long and composed of a scolex and three segments. The scolex has 30–36 hooks arranged in two rows. The first and second segments are incompletely developed while the last segment, which is gravid and contains up to 5000 ripe eggs, is half the length of the entire worm. dogs in towns are seldom affected but packs of hounds are commonly affected because of the method of feeding these dogs. The cystic stage is known as the echinococcus or hydatid cyst and gives rise to hydatid disease. It is found in cattle, sheep, pigs, deer and horses and can cause a serious and sometimes fatal disease in humans.

    Life cycle: After ripe ova are ingested by a suitable intermediate host, the capsules are dissolved by the digestive juices and the embryos penetrate through the wall of the small intestine. They enter the portal vein and some are retained in the liver, but others enter the systemic circulation and are spread to many varying situations in the body. The organs most commonly affected are the liver, lungs,

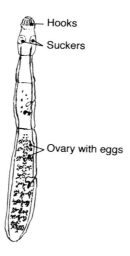

Fig. 16.2 *Echinococcus granulosus* (× 10).

kidneys and spleen. Occasionally cysts are found in the heart, bones and muscular tissue. The final host is the dog, which becomes infected by swallowing fertile cysts. As each cyst may contain hundreds of scolices, each of which is capable of developing into an adult worm, dogs can have a very heavy infestation. This is why echinococcus cysts are so common in the food animals.

The cyst has a fairly thick cuticle or capsule, which is concentrically laminated. It has an internal germinal layer. This layer produces numerous small vesicles or brood capsules about 5–6 months after infection and scolices are formed in these and on the germinal layer directly. Each brood capsule may contain up to 40 scolices invaginated into their neck portions and attached to the wall by stalks. The scolices and their stalks are covered by a cuticular layer. The brood capsules often become detached from the wall of the vesicle and float freely in the vesicular fluid, giving rise to the term 'hydatid sand'.

All echinococcus cysts do not form scolices. A large percentage are frequently sterile. In cattle 90% are sterile, in pigs about 20%, and in sheep about 8%. The sheep is therefore apparently the most suitable intermediate host. In cattle the cysts are often fibrotic.

Multiplication of the cyst can take place in various ways. Any factor that threatens the life of the cyst, e.g. entrance of bile, will lead to the formation of daughter cysts inside the original cyst, i.e. endogenous daughter cysts. These have a germinal layer and therefore can form scolices and grand-daughter cysts. Exogenous daughter cysts are formed by budding outwards, due to the escape of pieces of the germinal layer [Plate 5(d), (e)].

The cyst may burst into a body cavity, e.g. abdomen, and the scolices, brood capsules and germinal layer can all form new cysts.

Judgement: Affected parts are rejected.

Taenia hydatigena
This tapeworm occurs in the small intestine of the dog. It is a large worm up to 5 m in length. The scolex has 26–44 hooks in two rows.

Life cycle: The intermediate state is known as *Cysticercus tenuicollis*. This is found in the abdominal cavity of sheep, goat, deer, ox and pig. The cyst is one of the largest of the cysticerci, with a diameter of up to 7 cm. The neck is long and thin and the cyst is very often found hanging on the various organs and the periotoneum by the neck and not embedded in the tissues [Plate 2(a)].

When the eggs are swallowed by the intermediate host, the embryos hatch out in the intestine and pass through the intestinal wall. They reach the liver via the bloodstream and break out of the portal vessels. Occasionally they may pas into the posterior vena cava and be transported to other parts of the body. However, they usually burrow through the liver, causing the typical serpentine 'tenuicollis tracks' [Plate 6(F)], and eventually reach the liver surface. They then enter the abdominal cavity and the adult bladderworm may be found anywhere in the abdominal cavity lying in a delicvate cyst formed by the peritoneum. The cyst contains a watery fluid and a single white scolex invaginated into a long neck. The final host, i.e. the dog, becomes infected by ingesting the cysticercus. Sometimes small pea-size caseous and calcified degenerated cysts are found in the liver substance. Many lamb livers are affected.

Judgement: Usually the infection is a mild one and only requires removal of the cysts, but if the infection is extensive the organ or tissue should be rejected. This occurs most commonly with the omentum. Livers with haemorrhagic or degenerated 'tenuicollis tracks' should be rejected.

Taenia ovis

This tapeworm grows to about 1 m long, with a very small head with 24–36 hooks. It occurs in the small intestine of the dog. The intermediate stage, *Cysticercus ovis*, which measures 3–8 mm, is ovoid in form and contains a single scolex; it is found in the sheep and goat. The worms are usually found in the heart just under the epicardium [Plate 2(b)], but are also found in the diaphragm, skeletal muscles, tongue, masseter muscles and oesophagus. The cysts tend to degenerate early.

Life cycle: When the eggs are ingested by a sheep, the embryos hatch in the intestine, penetrate into the wall of the gut and reach the bloodstream, by which they are carried to the muscles. The cycle is completed with the dog eating affected muscle.

Judgement: Affected parts are rejected.

Multiceps multiceps

This occurs in the small intestine of the dog and is 40–100 cm long with a small head with 22–32 hooks.

Life cycle: The intermediate stage *Coenurus cerebralis* develops in the brain of ruminants, particularly sheep, producing a disease called 'gid' or 'sturdy'. The embryos, after hatching in the intestine, pass via the bloodstream to various parts of the body. Only those that reach the central nervous system develop. The young cysts travel about in the brain before settling down and are fully developed in 7–8 months. The fully grown cyst measures about 5 cm in diameter and has a delicate translucent wall that bears on its inner surface large numbers of scolices (up to several hundred). The dog becomes infected by eating affected brain tissue, and all or more of the fully formed scolices develop into tapeworms.

Symptoms of 'gid' may be shown in sheep at two different stages of infection. About 2 weeks after infection, when the embryos are wandering through the brain, the sheep may show symptoms of meningo-encephalitis such as nervousness or excitability. Acute cases may cause death in young lambs. Post-mortem examination of the brain then may show inflammation of the meninges and a number of yellowish sinuous tracks on the surface of the brain, at the ends of which the young bladderworms, about the size of a pin head, can be found. Such tracks may also be found in the heart and lungs.

This is succeeded about 6 months later by the chronic stage, which is associated with the increase in size of the cyst and the subsequent pressure atrophy of the brain substance. Affected animals may be blind, turn in circles or stagger (the typical 'giddy' sheep). The sheep are generally emaciated. On post-mortem examination one or more *Coenurus cerebralis* cysts are found on or in the brain, often lying in a cavity produced by pressure and are surrounded by necrotic material. There may be local pressure atrophy or perforation of the skull.

It should not be forgotten that the condition does occur in cattle and goats, although infrequently, with similar symptoms and results.

Judgement: In the early cases of 'gid' it is only necessary to reject the head, but in later stages the carcass should be rejected if it is emaciated.

Taenia pisiformis

This tapeworm of the dog is found in the small intestine and measures up to 2 mm in length, possessing 34–48 hooks on a small head. The intermediate stage is known as *Cysticercus pisiformis* and is found in rabbits and hares.

Life cycle: This is similar to *T. hydatigena*, but the intermediate hosts in this case are rabbits and hares. The young stages, after having developed in the veins of the liver for about a month, penetrate through the liver substance and the adult bladderworms are found in the abdominal cavity attached to the viscera. They are small cysts about the size of peas, as impled by the name *Cysticercus pisiformis*.

Judgement: Affected rabits and hares are generally thinner than normal but as the cysts are not found in the muscles only the affected organs should be rejected.

Multiceps serialis

This dog tapeworm is found in the small intestine and has a double row of 26–32 hooks; it may be up to 72 cm in length. The intermediate stage is known as *Coenurus serialis* and is found in the rabbit and sometimes in hares.

Life cycle: The eggs hatch in the intestine of the intermediate host, penetrate the gut wall, enter the bloodstream and are carried to the musculature. The common sites for the cysts are the intermuscular and subcutaneous tissue of the back, loin and hind limbs and not infrequently the muscles of the jaw. The cysts when fully developed may be up to 5 cm in diameter. They develop a number of scolices, which are invaginated into their necks. Internal as well as external daughter cysts may be found and these are also able to produce scolices.

The dog acquires the infection by eating the affected muscles.

The subcutaneous swellings caused by *Coenurus serialis* are obvious in the skinned or unskinned rabbits. When inspecting unskinned animals the hand should be carefully drawn from head to tail and the fluctuating cysts can be felt.

Judgement: Total rejection.

Tapeworms of humans

These are *Taenia saginata*, *T. solium* and *Diphyllobothrium latum* (extremely rare in Britain), and are found in the small intestine of humans as the result of eating affected flesh. They are therefore of importance in food inspection.

Taenia saginata

This occurs in the small intestine of humans whereas the intermediate stage *Cysticercus bovis* is found in cattle. The tapeworm measures from 4–10 m in length. The head has four elliptical suckers and to no hooks, and is said to be unarmed.

Life cycle: When the eggs are ingested by cattle, the embryos hatch in the intestine, penetrate the gut wall and reach the bloodstream by which they are carried to various parts of the body. The embryos that become lodged in the muscles develop into cysts – *Cysticercus bovis* – the so-called 'beef measles'.

Cysticercus bovis is first discernible about 2 weeks after infection as a solid white nodule but is clearly visible at 4 weeks. The mature cyst measures 9×5 mm and consists of a delicate, fluid-filled bladder surrounded by a fibrous capsule formed by the host [Plate 2(c)]. It is pinkish and the single scolex is seen as an opaque white spot. The cysts may remain viable for $1–2\frac{1}{2}$ years. The majority later undergo degeneration; changes from slight caseation to calcification are encountered.

The predilection sites for *Cysticercus bovis* are the masseter muscles, heart, tongue and the muscles of the shoulder and diaphragm, though cysts can occur in any muscle and in some organs, e.g. liver and lungs.

Humans become infected by eating affected undercooked beef.

The Fresh Meat (Hygiene and Inspection) Regulations 1995, Schedule 10, lay down methods of examination for *Cysticercus bovis* and the procedure that must be followed when found.

The methods of dissemination of the eggs are varied. Indiscriminate defaecation by the human host may result in the distribution of eggs or gravid segments on the land. Eggs may also be spread by sewage sludge or effluent, and it has been suggested that birds, particularly seagulls, may cause further spread by feeding on contaminated material.

Viability of a cyst may be demonstrated by incubating it at 37°C for half an hour in a solution of 30% of bile and 70% normal saline. If the cyst is viable, evagination of the head takes place.

Judgement: It is now the procedure when *Cysticercus bovis* is found, no matter at what stage, to reject the affected part and put the rest of the carcass and offal in cold store for 3 weeks at –7°C (20°F) or 14 days at –10°C (14°F). It is considered that if a cyst is found, this indicates infection and that other cysts are probably present.

Taenia solium

This tapeworm occurs in the small intestine of man and measures 3–8 m in length. The scolex has a double row of 26–28 hooks. The intermediate stage is called *Cysticercus cellulosae* and occurs in pigs, occasionally in humans and rarely in sheep and dog.

Life cycle: This is the same as *T. saginata*, but pigs act as the intermediary hosts. The cyst is of delicate structure and the invaginated scolex is seen as a pin-head-sized white spot. The size of *Cysticercus cellulosae* varies with its developmental stage from pin-head size up to 15×10 mm. It is elliptical in form. The cysts have a predilection for muscle although they can occur in the viscera. The muscles most commonly affected are those of the heart, diaphragm, tongue, neck and shoulder, and the intercostal and abdominal muscles. The cysts in pig may be scattered and few in number or they may be present in enormous numbers (up to 3000 cysts per 0.5 kg of muscle). Cysts tend to degenerate and become caseated and calcified.

Cysts may be detected during inspection 8 weeks after infection. They tend to degenerate and become caseated and calcified but, apart from sows and boars, pigs are generally slaughtered before these changes take place.

Judgement: Total rejection.

Diphyllobothrium latum

This tapeworm occurs in the small intestine and measures 2–10 m long. It has an oval, club-shaped head and has no hooklets. The final intermediate stage or *plerocercoid* occurs in freshwater fish.

Diphyllobothrium latum is extremely rare in Britain, if it occurs at all. However, one frequently encounters the plerocercoids of species of *Diphyllobothrium* from aquatic animals, such as seals, dolphins and porpoises and otters, in both salt and freshwater fish. They are harmless to humans.

Life cycle: The eggs develop for several weeks after leaving the body of the host, before the embryo is ready to hatch in water – the coracidium. This swims in the water and dies fairly quickly unless ingested by a suitable water flea or crustacean, e.g. *Cyclops strenuus* or *Diaptomus gracilis*.

In their body cavity a larval stage called a procercoid develops. If the crustacean is then swallowed by a suitable fish, the larval worm penetrates through the intestine to the muscle or other organs, where it develops into a plerocercoid. A large number of fish are known to act as secondary intermediate hosts, e.g. pike, salmon, trout and perch. The final host, i.e. humans, becomes infected through eating raw or insufficiently cooked fish or fish products.

In humans the worm produces severe anaemia, perhaps as the result of absorption of waste products or toxins.

Trematodes

These are known commonly as flukes. They are usually flat, leaf-shaped, parasitic worms without a body cavity, provided with a branched excretory sytem, and an alimentary canal usually without an anus, and are usually hermaphrodites. There are three trematodes of interest in meat inspection: *Fasciola hepatica* (Fig. 16.3) or common liver fluke, *Dicrocoelium dendriticum* and *Paramphistomum cervi*.

Fasciola hepatica

This is the common liver fluke. It is greyish brown in colour and reaches a size of

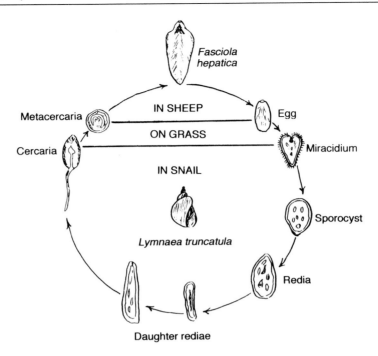

Fig. 16.3 Life cycle of *Fasciola*.

30 × 13 mm wide. It is leaf-shaped, broader anteriorly than posteriorly, with an anterior cone-shaped projection that is followed by a pair of broad 'shoulders'.

Life cycle: The adult worm lives in the bile ducts. The eggs enter the duodenum with the bile and leave the host in the faeces. Embryos or miracidia develop. They are actively motile but die soon unless they encounter a snail, *Lymnaea truncatula*. In the respiratory cavity of the snail they develop into sporocysts. Each sporocyst gives rise to 5–8 rediae. Daughter rediae may develop under unfavourable conditions but the next normal generation is one of cercariae. These leave the snail 4–7 weeks from the time of infection. Within minutes the cercariae settle on blades of grass and other plants just below water level and encyst there. At this stage they resemble grains of sand. One egg may give rise to over 300 cercariae. These may remain alive on pasture for up to a year. When grasses or other plants bearing encysted cercariae are eaten by grazing animals, the cysts are dissolved in the small intestine and the liberated embryos pass from the intestine to the liver and develop into adult flukes [Plate 2(e)]. Flukes can live in the liver for up to 10 years.

Sheep are more commonly infected than cattle, horses and deer because they graze the grass more closely and the majority of the cercariae encyst low down, particularly in marshy land. Liver fluke disease or distomatosis is connected with the life history of the snail *Lymnaea truncatula*, which starts to be active in March when it lays its eggs, the adult of which produces eggs 3 or 4 months later. Several generations are produced between March and October, thus there is a great increase in the snail population. Cercariae emerge from the liver of the snail early in Jul;y and outbreaks of acute fascioliasis occur in sheep in late August and early September. As *Fasciola hepatica* takes about 3 months to develop from the cercarial stage, the chronic form of the disease does not appear until late November or December. High rainfall in June increases the incidence of infection.

Post-mortem lesions: In acute cases there is acute swelling and congestion of the liver (acute hepatitis). This is due to the invasion of the liver by large numbers of young flukes. The capsule of the liver shows haemorrhages and is covered with fibrin. Section of the liver shows numerous circular holes from which emerge, when pressure is applied, necrotic liver tissue and immature flukes.

In chronic fascioliasis the liver in sheep becomes distorted and the bile ducts become enlarged, thickened and of a bluish colour. Flukes in a badly affected 'fluky' liver may number over 1000. Affected sheep carcasses are often emaciated and oedematous.

In cattle, in the chronic type, the liver becomes cirrhotic and the bile ducts become thickened, dilated and eventually calcified – the typical 'pipy' or 'fluky' liver.

In deer, infection is commonest in roe deer, in which it may be fatal. Other species have much more resistance. Cirrhosis is common but there is little reaction of the bile ducts (although they may contain many flukes), and therefore no 'pipy livers'.

It is interesting to note that small outbreaks occur in humans owing to consumption of watercress.

Animals in the wild are also affected, e.g. feral coypu in England.

Migratory flukes: In cattle, immature flukes may gain entrance to the bloodstream. Occasionally those flukes are found in cysts near the base of the lungs. The cyst is generally round, about 25 mm in diameter or slightly larger. In the early stages it contains the immature fluke and coagulated blood, but later it becomes calcified and contains a dark brown slime.

Flukes may also be found in the mesenteric nodes where they cause green caseous nodules, which are easily expressed from the lymph nodes. Similar lesions are caused in the mesenteric lymph nodes by *Linguatula serrata* larvae (p. 161).

Judgement: Affected organs are rejected. Affected sheep are often emaciated and oedematous. In such cases the judgement is total rejection.

Dicrocoelium dendriticum

This liver fluke is seldom found in this country, except in the west of Scotland, and is less pathogenic. The worm is slender, lance-shaped and very small, about 6–10 mm long by 2 mm wide. Up to 20 000 may be found in the liver. The life cycle is similar to that of *Fasciola hepatica* except that there are two intermediate hosts, a snail and an ant (*Formica fusta*).

Judgement: Reject liver.

Paramphistomum cervi
This is a pear-shaped fluke 5–13 mm long by 2–5 mm wide. It is light red in colour and occurs in the rumen and reticulum of sheep and cattle. The life cycle is very similar to that of *F. hepatica*.

The protozoa

These are single-celled organisms that are only visible microscopically. Multiplication takes place by division or budding. The protozoa important in meat inspection are coccidia (including toxoplasma), sarcocysts and haemosporidia.

Coccidia
The coccidia are parasites of the epithelium of the intestine and the bile ducts of mammals and birds. Two genera are found in domestic animals but only one is important in meat inspection, i.e. *Eimeria*. The typical life cycle of *Eimeria* is as follows.

The oöcyst containing eight sporozoites, which are contained in two sporocysts, is swallowed by the host and the sporozoites are liberated. Each enters a cell of the intestinal mucosa (or epithelial lining of the bile ducts) and grows at the expense of the cell. It is now called a trophozoite. It multiplies into 16 merozoites, which are liberated into the lumen. Each enters another cell and this asexual process is repeated. After some time a sexual cycle arises. A merozoite enters a cell, becomes a trophozoite and breaks up into a large number of comma-shaped forms. These are the male cells or microgametes, and the parent cell from which they arise is called the microgametocyte. Simultaneously another trophozoite in another cell forms a large single female cell or macrogamete. A microgamete enters a macrogamete and the zygote or oöcyst is formed. The oöcyst is passed in the faeces and its contents break up into sporoblasts and finally into sporocysts, when they are infective for another animal.

Coccidia of the *Eimeria* species cause intestinal disease (coccidiosis) in cattle, sheep, goats, rabbits and poultry. They may also be found in the liver of rabbits. Young animals of all species are more commonly affected and may scour severely and die. 'Shotty eruption' or 'Sooty mange' of the pig is said to be caused by a coccidium, but this is very doubtful.

Toxoplasma gondii, which is a coccidian parasite closely related to the genus *Isospora*, causes a disease called toxoplasmosis. Many animals are susceptible including humans, who are thought to be infected mainly from domestic cats. The disease causes abortion in sheep, which are thought to have become infected from straw bedding contaminated by cat faeces. Abortion also occurs in goats and probably deer. The fetal cotyledons show what are probably the characteristic lesions. The cotyledons are bright to dark red as compared with the normal deep purple and show numerous white flecks or nodules.

Judgement: Total rejection.

Sarcocysts

These are found encysted in the muscles and fasciae of cattle, sheep, pigs, deer and horses. They are oval-shaped structures, circular in cross-section and known as Miescher's tubes. They vary greatly in size from microscopic dimensions up to 10 mm in length. When they are easily visible to the naked eye. The Miescher's tubes are divided transversely into sections containing nucleated spores known as Rainey's corpuscles. The muscle cysts are yellowish white in colour. As they degenerate they become caseous and white and may eventually calcify.

The life cycle requires two hosts. Omnivorous animals, such as dogs, foxes and cats, ingest muscle cysts from herbivorous animals and pass the sporocysts in their faeces. Herbivorous animals ingest the sporocysts, which develop in the intestines and pass to the muscles. It is possible that blood-sucking and also non-blood-sucking flies may act as transport hosts. Over 35% of sheepdogs and up to 75% of hunting dogs have been found to be infected.

The cystic stages in the muscles are regarded as non-pathogenic but the earlier stages, which develop in the endothelium of blood vessels, may be very pathogenic, causing abortion in cattle and sheep, and may even prove to be fatal, particularly in calves,

Sarcocystis gigantea is the one most commonly found during meat inspection. It occurs in the muscle wall of the oesophagus of sheep and measures up to 1 cm in length. It is very much the largest sarcocyst found at meat inspection. Cats are the secondary hosts.

Sarcocystis tenella produces microscopic lesions in sheep. Dogs and foxes are the secondary hosts.

Sarcocystis ovicanis also affects sheep. It is found in cardiac muscle, skeletal muscle, spinal cord and fasciae, and massive numbers may be present. It is very much smaller than *S. gigantea* and measures about 3 mm in length. The secondary hosts are dogs and foxes. It is known that *S. ovicanis* is very pathogenic to sheep, which may adopt a dog-sitting position and be reluctant to stand.

Sarcocystis fusiformis (*S. cruzi*) affects cattle and is transmitted in the faeces of dogs and foxes. Cattle are also infected by *S. hominis*, which is transmitted in human faeces.

Sarcocystis miescheriana, S. suihominis and *S. porcifelis* affect pigs. *Sarcocystis miescheriana* has a pig–dog cycle whereas *S. porcifelis* has a pig–cat cycle and *S. suihominis* has a pig–human cycle.

Sarcocystis bertrami (*equicanis*) occurs in horses and has a horse–dog cycle. Over 60% of horses are affected. This high incidence indicates that many dogs must be fed on uncooked horse meat and offal. Infection can cause acute and chronic disease conditions.

Goats are infected by *S. capricornis, S. hiricanis* and *S. moulei*. The first two have a goat–dog cycle. The final host of *S. moulei* is unknown.

Sarcocystis wapati is found in the myocardium of deer. The lesions are microscopic. It is thought that a fox–deer or dog–deer cycle is involved.

Judgement: Dependent upon the degree of infestation, which can vary from a very few up to massive numbers of lesions. Total rejection when generalised infestation.

Haemosporidia

These organisms are parasitic in the bloodstream and are transmitted by blood-sucking ticks or flies. The only one of importance in meat inspection in the UK is *Babesia divergens*.

Babesia divergens causes red-water (babesiasis) in cattle. Infection is spread by the tick *Ixodes ricinus*. Post-mortem findings are: enlarged liver and spleen, jaundice, anaemia and haemoglobin-stained urine in bladder.

Judgement: Depends upon state of carcass.

Arthropoda

With the exception of the 'sheep head fly' (*Hydrotaea irritans*) and the sheep ked (*Melophagus ovinus*), adult flies are of little importance in meat inspection, but in several the larval stage is. These are warble flies (*Hypoderma bovis* and *H. lineatum*), sheep nostril fly (*Oestrus ovis*), deer nasal flies (*Cephenemyia aur-ibarbua* and *C. stimulator*), horse bots (*Gastrophilus intestinalis*) and sheep maggot fly (*Lucilia sericata*).

There are other flies not dealt with here that can annoy and irritate animals. These can be separated into two groups: biting flies and nuisance flies, e.g. stable fly, horn fly, cattle biting fly, blackfly, horse-fly, cleg, head fly, face fly, cattle sweat fly and the ordinary house fly.

Hypoderma bovis, H. lineatum, H. diana, H. aeratum and Przhevalskiana silenus (warble flies)

These are large, two-winged insects with hairy bodies. There are two species of importance, *Hypoderma bovis* (Fig. 16.4) and *H. lineatum*. The hairs on the head and anterior part of the thorax are greenish yellow in *H. bovis* and yellowish white in *H. lineatum*. The abdomen is covered with light yellow hairs anteriorly, followed by a band of dark hairs, and the posterior portion bears orange–yellow hairs.

Hypoderma diana affects deer. Very heavy infestations can occur in deer in the wild. Occasionally extensive and severe negrosis occurs in the subcutaneous tissue and muscles owing to secondary infection by *Corynebacterium pyogenes*. Losses can be severe.

Gadding does not occur as in cattle.

Sheep are occasionally affected by *H. diana* but only when they are in close contact with deer.

Hypoderma eratum and *Przhevalskiana silenus* affect goats.

Life cycle: The flies occur in the summer and are most active on warm days, when they attack the cattle to lay their eggs. These are about 1 mm long and are

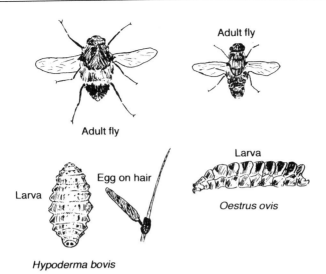

Fig. 16.4 *Hypoderma bovis* and *Oestrus ovis*.

fixed to the hairs by means of small terminal clasps, especially on the legs, but more rarely on the body. *Hypoderma bovis* lays its eggs singly while *H. lineatum* deposits a row or more on a hair. The flies are very persistent in attacking the animals, and one female may lay 100 or more eggs on one animal. The eggs hatch in a few days and the larvae crawl down the hair and penetrate the skin. They wander up the subcutaneous tissue of the leg and then to the diaphragm. The larvae of *H. lineatum* are often found in the oesophageal wall (where they cause an odema of the wall) from the end of December to mid-February, when they measure 12 mm in length. In the latter part of the winter the larvae travel towards the dorsal aspect of the body and reach the subcutaneous tissue of the back. The larvae of *H. bovis* sometimes enter the spinal canal but usually leave it again. When the parasites arrive under the skin, swellings begin to form, measuring about 3 cm in length. The skin over each swelling becomes perforated and the larvae are able to breathe. They become noticeable on the back as nodules from February to May, being visible for about a month before they emerge from the back to pupate on the ground. The adult flies emerge about 1 month later. The complete life cycle therefore takes 1 year. The younger larvae are almost white, changing to yellow and then to light brown as they grow older. The full grown larva measures about 28 mm long.

When the flies approach to lay eggs the cattle become scared and try to escape by running away, often with their tails in the air ('gadding') and even go into water. Since the flies are persistent, the animals are constantly irritated and do not feed properly, which results in loss of weight and decrease of milk yield. The larvae irritate the tissues around them and the flesh becomes greenish yellow and infiltrated, 'licked back'. Inflammatory changes may be produced in the spinal canal and oesophageal wall. Great damage is caused to the skin by the perforations produced [Plate 6(e)]. Calves and young cattle are more frequently and more severely infested than older animals.

Judgement: Local trimming of affected back fat is sufficient.

Oestrus ovis (sheep nostril fly, Fig. 16.4)

The adult fly deposits larvae upon the nostrils of the sheep. They crawl up the nasal passages and sinuses and feed upon the exudates produced by their irritant action. When fully developed the larvae measure 3 cm in length and 60–80 may be present in the nasal cavities. A heavy infestation causes a mucopurulent nasal discharge.

Judgement: Reject affected heads.

Cephenemyia auribarbua and C. stimulator (deer nasal flies)

The life cycles and conditions caused are similar to those of the sheep nostril fly in sheep.

Judgement: Reject affected heads.

Gastrophilus intestinalis (horse bot fly)

This is similar to the warble flies and lays eggs on the horse's body. Owing to licking, the larvae are ingested and penetrate the mucosa of the mouth and eventually reach the stomach where they attach to the oesophageal portion. The fully developed larvae are about 3 cm in length, resembling warbles, and large numbers may be found attached to the stomach. They remain there for about 10 months, when they are passed out in the faeces to pupate and hatch on the ground.

Judgement: Reject stomach.

Lipoptena cervi (deer ked)

The adult emerges from the pupa on the ground, takes wing and lands on the deer. The wings break off and the fly spends the rest of its life on the deer. Although they may be very numerous they seem to cause little damage.

Melophagus ovinus (sheep ked)

This is a small wingless fly that sucks blood and spends its entire life on sheep. Its irritant bite can result in sores, which attract other flies. If abundant, anaemia may ensue.

Deer may also be affected.

Judgement: Based on degree of anaemia.

Lucilia sericata (sheep maggot fly)

The adult fly deposits larvae on sheep, producing maggoty or 'fly blown' sheep. Affected animals are not often seen in meat inspection, but where there is evidence of maggot infection, extensive trimming may be necessary as the larvae can burrow deeply into the muscle tissue. Chronic abscesses may result from the activities of the larvae and these are most often found in the hind-quarters.

Judgement: Reject affected parts.

Hydrotaea irritans (sheep head fly)

Intense irritation is caused to sheep by this non-biting fly causing 'sheep head fly disease'. The results are wounded or 'broken' heads. It is common in the border counties of Scotland and England. The fly is like the common house fly but with an olive-green abdomen and orange–yellow wing bases. It is associated with forestry plantations and is active in July and August. Large swarms feed on nose and eye secretions causing the sheep to rub their heads on undergrowth and fences or scratch with their hind feet. Breeds of sheep without a lot of wool about their heads are the most susceptible.

In deer the flies cause irritation to stags 'in velvet' and prevent them from grazing and resting properly.

The fly also spreads summer mastitis in cattle.

Judgement: Reject head.

Contamination of meat by Arthropoda larvae

The larvae or maggots occasionally found on meat belong to the bluebottles or blowflies, e.g. *Calliphora vomitoria* or *C. erythrocephela*. The adult flies lay their eggs on the meat and these hatch in a few hours or days. The larvae continue to grow for about 10 days before pupating.

'Fly blown' means having had fly eggs laid upon it. 'Fly strike' indicates successful establishments of maggots.

The larvae of the ham beetle, *Dermestes lardarius* is 6–10 mm long with a wide pale-yellow band across its back.

The flour mite or *Tyroglyphus farinae* may be seen in meat.

Linguatula serrata

A pentastome closely related to the spiders, ticks and mites. It is important in meat inspection because the larvae are found in the mesenteric lymph nodes of cattle, sheep, horse and rabbit. The lesions produced are very similar to those of tuberculosis.

Life cycle: The adult lives in the nasal cavity of the dog for about 2 years. Eggs first appear in the nasal discharge 6 months after infection and may number up to half a million. When the ova are ingested by cattle, the embryos are conveyed by the blood and lymph stream to the mesenteric lymph nodes, but may be found in the liver and lungs or any other part of the body. The larvae are 6–10 mm long and are chiefly found in cattle but also in sheep, pig and rabbit.

The larval forms (commonly called pentastomes) are seen in the mesenteric nodes as small nodules about the size of a millet seed or pea, usually at the periphery of the nodes and which shell out easily. The lesions are greenish or grey in colour and are soft but eventually may calcify. In the early stages the larvae can be seen in the lesions, but later only the typical chitinous hooks may be seen microscopically. Dogs become infected by eating infected rabbits or nodes of large animals.

Judgement: Reject affected parts.

Lice (Fig. 16.5)

These are flat wingless insects that infest animals and birds. Some exist on skin debris, others by biting and sucking the blood of the host. The host is apt to lose condition when badly infected because of irritation caused by the lice. The commonest species affecting animals are *Trichodectes, Haematopinus, Damalinia* and *Linognathus.*

Damalinia ovis is a biting louse that feeds on skin debris and is found mainly on the back and neck of sheep.

Haematopinus ovillus, which sucks blood, is found on the body of sheep.

Judgement: Dependent on the state of the carcass.

Mecanthus stramineus (body louse) and *Liponyssus caponis* (wing louse) affect poultry. *M. stramineus* also affects turkeys.

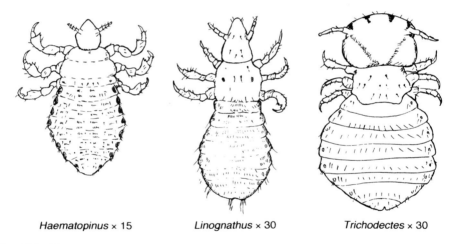

Haematopinus × 15   Linognathus × 30   Trichodectes × 30

Fig. 16.5   Lice.

Mites or Acaridae (Fig. 16.6)

These cause mange in animals and man. There are four types of mange: sarcoptic, psoroptic, horioptic and demodectic.

Judgement: In all cases of mange, judgement depends upon the severity of the lesions and the state of the carcass.

Sarcoptes scabiei

This is a minute parasite, roughly circular in outline, characterised by the pre-

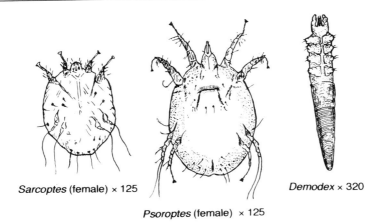

Sarcoptes (female) × 125   Demodex × 320

Psoroptes (female) × 125

Fig. 16.6   Mites.

sence of suckers with unjointed pedicles on the first two pairs of legs in the male and female and on the fourth pair in males.

Life cycle: The female burrows in the skin and lays 20–40 eggs. The larvae hatch in a few days and have three pairs of legs. A nymphal stage, with four pairs of legs, follows, which gives rise to males or females. The whole life cycle is believed to take 2–3 weeks.

All animals can be affected by sarcoptic mange but it is commonest in pigs, particularly sows, and cattle. The skin becomes inflamed and swollen, and dry; scurfy areas are characteristic. Constant rubbing owing to the irritation results in the formation of raw areas and of large scales and cracks from which blood and serum exude. Animals suffering from the moist form of the disease often have a very offensive smell and the skin later becomes wrinkled and thrown into folds. Emaciation becomes a marked feature.

Sarcoptic mange is a notifiable disease of horses.

Psoroptes

This genus contains a number of parasites that live on different hosts and, contrary to sarcoptes, are specific for their host.

The psoroptes are larger and longer than the sarcoptes. Their legs, which project beyond their bodies, have suckers with jointed pedicles. The most important psoropte is *Psoroptes communis ovis*, which causes *sheep scab*, a notifiable disease.

The mites puncture the epidermis to suck lymph and cause small inflammatory swellings infiltrated with serum. This exudes onto the surface and coagulates forming a crust. The wool becomes loose and falls out or it is pulled out by the sheep biting and scratching. The diseased condition of the skin and the constant irritation lead to progressive emaciation.

Psoroptic mange is a notifiable disease of horses.

Chorioptes

These cause a similar lesion to psoroptic mange but are confined to the legs and belly. Cattle, horses and sheep are affected. The species of this genus are named after the hosts, e.g. *Chorioptes bovis, C. equi* and *C. ovis.*

Demodex

This is a very specialised group of parasitic mites that live in the hair follicles and sebaceous glands of the skin, causing *demodectic* or *follicular mange* in nearly all animals.

The parasites are elongated, usually about 0.25 mm long and have a head, a thorax which bears four pairs of stumpy legs, and an elongated abdomen. Most species are named after the hosts, e.g. *D. equi, D. bovis, D. ovis* and *D. caprae.* The pig is affected by *D. phylloides.*

Two forms of the disease are usually recognised. In the scaly form there is loss of hair, and thickening and wrinkling of the skin. The skin becomes scaly and is usually reddened.

The pustular form is due to bacterial invasion and is usually preceded by the scaly form. Pustules a few millimetres in diameter develop, or large abscesses may form. Itching is not so severe as in other forms of mange.

In cattle the neck, shoulders and back regions are mainly affected with the scaly type. Sheep are seldom affected and if so it is generally by the scaly form, whereas in goats the pustular form is the most common. In the pig large abscesses may form.

Ticks

Ticks are the most important external parasites of animals, especially in hot countries. They are the carriers of many diseases and are closely related to mites. In the UK the only tick of importance is *Ixodes ricinus* (sheep or castor bean tick) (Fig. 16.7). The life cycle lasts 3 years and it is a three-host tick. The three hosts are attacked by the nymph, the larva and the adult. Each stage leaves its host and moults on the ground. The three hosts may be of different species of animal. The adult tick imbeds its head and sucks blood. The feamel may treble in size on engorging blood. The male does not increase in size.

In cattle it causes babesiasis (see p. 158) and tick-borne fever.

In sheep it causes tick-borne fever and tick pyaemia.

Three types of ticks are found on deer: *Ixodes ricinus*, which is the commonest, *Dermacentor reticulatus* and *Haemaphysalis punctata.*

Moulds

A few moulds are found on meat, particularly imported chilled or frozen meat. There are four moulds (Fig. 16.8) that are important:

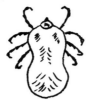

Fig. 16.7   *Ixodes ricinus* (engorged female, × 2).

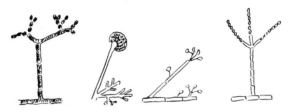

Cladosporium   Thamnidium   Sporotrichum   Penicillium

Fig. 16.8   Moulds.

(1)   *Cladosporium herbarum* – 'black spot' [Plate 4(e)]
(2)   *Sporotrichum carnis* – 'white spot'
(3)   *Thamnidium* – 'whiskers'
(4)   *Penicillium* – 'blue-green mould'.

Moulds have a typical unpleasant mouldy or musty taste and smell. Most of them, however, are non-toxic. A few do produce dangerous toxins, e.g. *Aspergillus flavus* on cereals and groundnuts. It produces a toxin, *aflatoxin*, that causes a serious and often fatal disease in poultry fed on contaminated foodstuff.

Cladosporium herbarum
This is the mould that causes 'black spot'. It is frequently found in imported chilled and frozen beef and mutton. In beef, the black spots, which are about 5 mm in diameter, are commonly found on the neck, skirt and pleura and, in frozen mutton, on the legs and in the thoracic and abdominal cavities. 'Black spot' cannot be removed by scraping or wiping as it penetrates into the meat.
   Judgement: It may be possible to trim if the infection is very slight but total rejection is generally the case.

Sporotrichum carnis
This is the mould that causes small, flat, woolly, 'white spots' on imported meat. It grows on the surface of the meat and can generally be removed by wiping.
   Judgement: If slight it may be wiped off.

Thamnidium

This causes 'whiskers' on meat and is superficial in its growth.

   Judgement: It may be wiped off if slight.

Penicillium

This is a bluish-green mould and is a superficial growth.

   Judgement: Wipe off if slight.

Parasitic fungi

Ringworm in animals, including humans, is caused by various types of fungi. It is probably the commonest zoonosis affecting personnel in slaughterhouses and because of this the lesions should not be handled. Cattle can be symptomless carriers of the fungal spores on their skin.

   The typical lesion consists of a circumscribed, elevated patch on the skin that becomes covered with scabs or scales and may or may not be denuded of hair. It is especially common in young animals, particularly calves, caused by *Trichophyton verrucosum*. It occasionally affects sheep. The lesions are most commonly found about the head, face, lips, eyelids and neck.

   Trichophyton metagrophytes can cause ringworm lesions up to 15 cm in diameter on the skin of the face, shoulders and flanks of sows.

   Aspergillus fumigatus causes aspergillosis. The fungus is common in mouldy hay and straw. The spores invade the tissues or colonise body cavities, causing various diseases, e.g. mycotic abortion in cattle, mycotic pneumonia of deer and aspergillosis in poultry (see p. 262).

Chapter 17
Affections of Specific Parts and Tumours

It is important to remember that tumours and abscesses can occur in any organ or tissue.

Blood

Anaemia

This may be defined as a deficiency in blood owing to haemorrhage or blood-sucking worms and parasites, or a deficiency of blood pigment, or a decrease in the number of red blood corpuscles that may be the result of some chronic disease, e.g. Jöhne's disease. Anaemia is not easy to detect in the live animal other than by pallid mucous membranes and breathlessness. An anaemic carcass is generally pale in colour, is often emaciated and sets poorly.

Judgement: The carcass and offal are rejected.

Jaundice or icterus

Details of these affections are given in Chapter 14.

Uraemia

This occurs when there is obstruction to the normal outflow of urine from the body. The result is that the blood has a smell of urine that is transmitted to all the organs and tissues. Urinary calculi are the commonest cause of this condition, occurring mainly in rams and boars. Hydronephrosis and pyelonephritis are other conditions in which uraemia may develop.

Judgement: Carcasses affected with uraemia are rejected. In case of doubt the boiling test is useful (p. 102). Rupture of the bladder at slaughter resulting in contamination of the peritoneum gives a strong urinous smell in the abdominal cavity. In these cases stripping of the peritoneum may be all that is necessary.

Leukaemia (see enzootic bovine leukosis, p. 125)

This is a chronic disease in which there is an increase in the number of white blood corpuscles. Proliferative changes may occur in the bone marrow – myeloid leukaemia, or in the lymph nodes and spleen – lymphatic leukaemia, which is the commoner type. Old cows are the most commonly affected, followed by pigs and sheep. In affected animals the lymph nodes and spleen are enlarged and characteristic lymphatic tissue lesions or tumours are found in various organs, particularly liver and kidneys. The condition is now called lymphosarcoma.

Judgement: Total rejection.

Hydraemia

In this condition the blood is more watery and is thinner than normal blood. Hydraemic carcasses are somewhat like oedematous carcasses but appear almost as if they had been soaked in water. The associated fluid is more watery than oedematous fluid. The condition is common in old ewes with chronic fascioliasis.

Judgement: Carcasses should be detained for 24 hours before judgement, to see if they dry out.

Haemoglobinaemia

This is caused by the accumulation of haemoglobin in the blood plasma owing to the rapid destruction of large numbers of red blood corpuscles. Evidence is seen in the urine, which turns red – haemoglobinuria. It occurs in certain diseases, e.g. red-water of cattle (p. 158) and azoturia of horses (p. 118).

Judgement: Dependent upon the state of the carcass.

Hypocalcaemia

This is a condition in which there is a decrease in the amount of calcium in the blood, e.g. milk fever in cows and transit tetany. There are no diagnostic post-mortem lesions in such cases but animals so affected may bleed and set badly and may be badly bruised from being recumbent for long periods.

Judgement: Dependent upon the state of the carcass.

Hypomagnesaemia

This is a condition in which there is a decrease in the amount of magnesium in the blood. Cattle so affected are often found dead. There are no diagnostic post-mortem lesions but animals slaughtered while so affected may bleed badly.

Judgement: Dependent upon the state of the carcass.

Bone

Bones of the bovine

(1) Fractures – especially ribs, pelvic and leg bones. 'Split aitches' or fractures in the region of the pubic symphysis are a fairly common occurrence when animals slip and splay their hind legs. Old fractures that have healed with callus formation are common in the ribs.

(2) Actinomycosis (p. 116).

(3) Tuberculosis – vertebrae most commonly (p. 135).

(4) Melanosis (p. 107).

(5) Presternal calcification in the brisket (putty brisket). See p. 194. This is a pressure necrosis owing to bruising during lying down. It is not a bone condition but is a fat necrosis [Plate 6(c)], and irregular putty-like masses develop and eventually calcify. It can be confused with tuberculosis but may be distinguished by the lustreless dead-white colour, by not being in the bone, and by the absence of tuberculous lesions in associated lymph nodes, i.e. the presternal and suprasternal nodes.

Judgement: It is a local condition and only requires trimming of affected part.

(6) Rickets in young animals. It is characterised by softening, swelling and curvature of the bones and is caused by deficiency of vitamin D or sunlight.

Judgement: Total rejection.

(7) Osteomalacia. This is a bone disease of the adult. It is caused by decalcification of the bones. This may be so pronounced that only a thin shell of bone remains. The periosteum is easily peeled off the bone and the bone marrow is of a dark-red jelly-like consistency. This is most easily seen in the sawn vertebrae and sternum.

Judgement: Total rejection.

(8) Osteohaematochromatosis (p. 108): brown pigmentation of bones of calf.

(9) *Echinococcus* cysts – rare (p. 148).

(10) Tumours, especially sarcomata (p. 192).

Judgement: Total rejection.

Bones of sheep

(1) Fractures

(2) Melanosis (p. 107).

Bones of pigs

(1) Fractures, especially ribs and 'split aitches', which is commonest in pigs.

Judgement: Reject affected parts.

(2) Rickets.

Judgement: Total rejection.

(3)   Tuberculosis, especially vertebrae, ribs and femur (p. 135).

(4)   Abscesses (p. 104), particularly in vertebrae as a complication of damaged tails ('Tail biting', p. 187).

(5)   Ossifying spondylitis (ankylosing spondylosis). This is a condition in which the various ligaments of the vertebrae undergo progressive ossification (exostosis) with resulting rididity of the backbone. It is not uncommon in adult sows, affecting the thoracic and lumbar regions. It is of little importance in meat inspection. Bulls and adult sheep may also be affected.

(6)   Osteohaematochromatosis (p. 108).

Head and tongue

Bovine head and tongue

(Bovine head is SBM and will be rejected anyway.)

(1)   Actinobacillosis (p. 115)
(2)   Actinomycosis (p. 116).
(3)   Foot and mouth disease (p. 125).
(4)   Calf diphtheria (p. 123).
(5)   Tuberculosis affecting lymph nodes (p. 135).
(6)   Ringworm (p. 166).
(7)   *Cysticercus bovis* (p. 152).
(8)   Melanosis (p. 107).
(9)   Xanthosis (p. 108).
(10)   Abscesses in tonsils (p. 104).
(11)   Bovine virus diarrhoea (p. 123).
(12)   Malignant catarrhal fever (p. 130).

Sheep head and tongue

(1)   Orf (p. 130).
(2)   Larvae of *Oestrus ovis* (p. 160).
(3)   *Coenurus cerebralis* (p. 150).
(4)   Foot and mouth disease (p. 125).
(5)   Sheep head fly disease (p. 161).
(6)   Drenching gun injuries to the pharynx.
       Judgement: Reject affected parts.
(7)   Ringworm (p. 166).
(8)   Actinobacillosis (p. 115).
(9)   Actinomycosis (p. 116).
(10)   Lice (p. 162).

Pig head and tongue

(1)   Tuberculosis (p. 135).

(2)   *Corynebacterium equi* lesions in lymph nodes. These lesions may be confused with those of avian tuberculosis. They are small, white necrotic lesions that are surrounded by connective tissue capsules and can be 'shelled' out easily. The necrotic tissue sometimes has the appearance and consistency of white lead paint.
   Judgement: Remove affected lymph nodes.

(3)   Foot and mouth disease (p. 125).

(4)   Swine vesicular disease (p. 135).

(5)   Anthrax (p. 116).

(6)   Abscesses. These are common affecting the submaxillary, parotid and retropharyngeal regions and their lymph nodes (p. 104).
   Judgement: Reject head only if no further spread.

(7)   Oedema of the eyelids in bowel oedema.
   Judgement: Reject head.

(8)   Atrophic rhinitis. In this condition the snout becomes dished and there is wrinkling of the skin over the affected area. The turbinate bones show atrophy, congestion and areas of necrosis. The nasal septum is distorted and there is often a bloody, nasal discharge. *Pasteurella multocida* causes a severe type of disease and *Bordetella bronchiseptica* a milder type.
   Judgement: Reject head and check for systemic infections such as septicaemia, pyaemia and toxaemia.

(9)   Damage to ears, e.g. bites and haematoma when the auricle of the ear is ballooned and full of blood.
   Judgement: Trim off affected ear.

(10)   Ringworm (p. 166).
   Judgement: Reject head.

Deer head and tongue

(1)   Actinomycosis (p. 115).

(2)   Foot and mouth disease (p. 125).

(3)   Gun-shot wounds (p. 6).

(4)   Tuberculosis of lymph nodes (p. 135).

(5)   Maglignant catarrhal fever (p. 130).

(6)   Nasal flies (p. 160).

(7)   *Hydrotaea irritans* (p. 161).

(8)   Lice (p. 162).

Heart

Bovine heart

(1) Pericarditis (inflammation of the pericardium). Characterised by the pericardial sac adhering to the heart wall, and the serous membranes becoming opaque.

    (a) Traumatic. This is generally due to a piece of wire or nail that has been swallowed, lodged in the reticulum and has penetrated the wall of the reticulum, diaphragm and the pericardium. The result is a fibrinous or septic pericarditis. Very often there is found in association a septic or gangrenous pneumonia. The foreign body may actually pass from the abdomen into the thorax and be found embedded in the heart or lungs. A fistulous tract can often be found. Toxaemia may result.

    (b) Tuberculous (p. 135).

    (c) Simple non-specific.

        Judgement: Total rejection when acute septic pericarditis, otherwise reject heart.

(2) Epicardial haemorrhages, e.g. septicaemia.

    Judgement: Reject heart.

(3) *Cysticercus bovis* in myocardium (heart muscle) (p. 152).

(4) Pyaemic abscesses in myocardium.

    Judgement: Total rejection.

(5) Xanthosis (p. 108).

(6) Endocarditis (inflammation of the endocardium). In almost all cases this is confined to the heart valves and most cases are bacterial in origin, e.g. ulcerative valvular endocarditis is sometimes seen in calves and older cattle and this is caused by streptococci or *Corynebacterium pyogenes*.

    Judgement: Reject heart.

(7) Melanosis (p. 107).

(8) Jaundice. This shows up particularly well on the fat of the heart (p. 107).

(9) *Echinococcus* cysts (p. 148).

(10) Brown atrophy (p. 105)

(11) Periarteritis nodosa (polyarteritis). This is a rare condition. Nodular fibrous thickenings occur along the branches of the coronary artery and are circular on cross-section.

(12) Listeriosis (p. 129).

Sheep heart

(1) *Cysticercus ovis* (p. 150).

(2) Pericarditis (see above).

(3)   Myocarditis [inflammation of the heart muscle (myocardium)].
(4)   Sarcocysts (p. 157).
(5)   Melanosis (p. 107).
(6)   *Echinococcus* cysts (p. 148).
(7)   Blood splashing especially in lambs (pp. 83, 180).
      Judgement: In all cases reject the hearts.

Pig heart

(1)   Pericarditis. Septic and fibrinous in swine erysipelas (p. 133).
(2)   Epicarditis (inflammation of the epicardium).
(3)   Endocarditis.
(4)   Verrucose endocarditis (swine erysipelas (p. 133).
(5)   Petechial haemorrhages, e.g. swine fever (p. 134).
(6)   Sarcocysts (p. 157).
      Judgement: In all cases reject heart.

Joints

Bovine joints

(1)   Arthritis or inflammation of the joint:

  (a)   Acute septic arthritis, which occurs in calves with umbilical infection – 'joint ill' in calves. This type of arthritis also occurs as a complication in cows with septic metritis.
  (b)   Septic arthritis occurs in joints of the foot of cattle with 'foul of the foot'.
  (c)   Chronic arthritis.
  (d)   Polyarthritis is when numerous joints are affected by a blood-borne infection. The commonest bacteria involved are streptococci, staphylococci, *Bacteroides necrophorus. Haemophilus* and *Chlamydia psittaci.*
        Judgement: Total rejection if evidence of systemic infections such as septicaemia, pyaemia and toxaemia or emaciation found, otherwise reject affected parts.

(2)   Rheumatism. This is characterised by thickening of tissues and enlargement of the joint.
      Judgement: Total rejection if evidence of systemic infections such as septicaemia, pyaemia and toxaemia or emaciation found, otherwise reject affected parts.

(3)   Dislocation.
      Judgement: Reject affected parts.

Sheep joints

(1) Arthritis – especially chronic arthritis affecting stifle and fetlock joints.
(2) Polyarthritis caused by *B. necrophorus*, *Haemophilus agni* and *C. psittaci*.
   Judgement: As bovine.

Pig joints

(1) Arthritis, e.g. in chronic swine erysipelas (p. 133), Glässer's disease (p. 127) and in *Mycoplasma hyosynoviae* infection. In these conditions polyarthritis is common.
   Judgement: As bovine.
(2) Rheumatism.
   Judgement: As bovine.
(3) Dislocations. It is important to distinguish between ante-and post-mortem dislocations. Frequently, post-mortem dislocation of the elbow joint particularly occurs in the dehairing machine. As the animal has been bled and the heart has stopped beating, no bruising takes place, as opposed to the bruising that occurs with ante-mortem dislocation.
   Judgement: If ante-mortem reject affected part.

Kidneys

Bovine kidneys

(1) Nephritis – acute and chronic [Plate 3(c)]. Infection of the kidney which may be caused by bacterial infection, viral infection, toxins or poisons.
   Judgement: Check for uraemia (p. 167) and reject kidney.
(2) Hydronephrosis – caused by obstruction to the outflow of urine. The ureter of the kidney is dilated and the pressure may lead eventually to the obliteration of kidney tissue with the formation of large thin-walled cysts containing urine [Plate 3(b)].
   Judgement: Check for uraemia (p. 167) and reject kidneys.
(3) Multiple congenital cysts – usually bilateral and grain-sized, and irregularly distributed throughout the kidneys.
   Judgement: Reject kidneys.
(4) Petechial haemorrhages, e.g. in septicaemia or toxaemia (p. 111).
(5) Pyaemic abscesses (p. 000).
(6) Infarcts. These are caused by non-pyogenic emboli becoming lodged in the renal capillaries. They lead to necrosis of the kidney tissue surrounding the embolism. They are pyramidal or wedge-shaped with their bases situated at the kidney surface.
   Judgement: Reject kidneys and check for cause.

(7) Pyelonephritis. Most commonly seen in cows as an ascending infection from bladder, etc. It is an infection of the renal pelvis by pyogenic organisms. It may be uni-or bilateral. The pelvis is filled with a slimy, gairy fluid intermixed with pus. It has a strong smell of ammonia. The ureters are generally much enlarged and contain similar fluid. Very often there are abscesses in the kidney substance and irregular yellowish or greenish-grey areas on the kidney surface. Uraemia and oedema of the cardass may develop.

    Judgement: Local rejection if very slight but generally there is total rejection.

(8) Fibroplastic nephritis or 'white spotted kidney' is found in calves. It is a form of non-suppurative interstitial nephritis that regresses as the calf grows older. It may be caused by *E. coli*. The surface of the kidney shows numerous white nodules up to 8 mm in diameter. They are circular or wedge-shaped in cross-section and are confined to the cortex of the kidney [Plate 6(b)].

    Judgement: Reject kidneys.

(9) Tuberculosis. This is a haematogenous spread and usually shows as small caseous nodules but also whole lobes may be affected (p. 135).

    Judgement: Reject kidney and suprarenal gland.

(10) Hypernephroma – this is a tumour that occurs on the anterior part of the kidney that is in contact with the suprarenal gland. Other kinds of tumours are also found in the kidneys, e.g. lymphosarcoma.

    Judgement: This depends upon the number of other tumours present in the offal and carcass and their type.

Sheep kidneys

These can show all the affections that occur in bovine kidneys with the exceptions of fibroplatic nephritis and tuberculosis, which are very rare in sheep. Pyaemic abscesses are commoner in sheep kidneys than in those of the other animals.

Pig kidneys

(1) Petechial haemorrhages – e.g. swine fever and swine erysipelas (pp. 133 and 134).

(2) Infarcts (p. 174).

(3) Verrucae, which are special types of infarcts that occur in chronic swine erysipelas (p. 133).

(4) Nephritis. The chronic type is fairly common in pigs' kidneys, which are pale in colour and have a hard, pitted surface; the capsule is firmly attached.

    Judgement: As bovine.

(5) Hydronephrosis.

    Judgement: As bovine.

(6) Congenital cysts, which are small and usually very numerous.
     Judgement: As bovine.
(7) Pyelonephritis. It has been found that water shortage resulting from frozen pipes can be a contributory factor.
     Judgement: Total rejection.
(8) *Stephanurus dentatus* (p. 146).
     Judgement: Reject kidneys.

Deer kidneys

(1) Congenital cysts.
     Judgement: As bovine.
(2) Hydronephrosis.
     Judgement: As bovine.
(3) Nephritis.
     Judgement: As bovine.
(4) Kidney stones.
     Judgement: Reject kidneys.

Liver

Bovine Liver

(1) Hepatitis (inflammation of the liver). Caused by bacterial or viral infection, parasite infestation, toxins, poisons or pesticides.
     Judgement: Reject liver and investigate cause.
(2) Peritonitis (p. 188).
(3) Fatty change:

     (a) Physiological – seen in high-yielding dairy cows in early lactation and also in cows in late pregnancy on inadequate diets. Liver remains firm to the touch.
          Judgement: Fit, but may be rejected on aesthetic grounds.
     (b) Pathological – nucleus of the liver cells is destroyed, therefore liver is greasy and friable to the touch. Caused by septicaemia or toxaemia.
          Judgement: Reject liver and check other organs.

(4) Telangiectasis, or cavernous haemangioma or angioma. This occurs in the livers of adult animals of all species but particularly in the livers of old cows. It shows as bluish black depressed areas of irregular shape with well defined edges scattered throughout the liver substances. They vary in size ferom 1 to 3 mm and are clearly see through the serous capsule of the liver. When cut through they appear as sponge-like areas from which blood exudes or which can be easily expressed. The cause is unknown.
     Judgement: Dependent upon the degree of affection.

(5)   Tumours. The liver is a common site of tumours (p. 192).

(6)   Bacterial necrosis, bacillary necrosis or necrobacillosis caused by *Bacteroides necrophorus*. This is considered to be spread from lesions in the rumen. The lesion can be in various forms, e.g. in the form of an abscess (common in 'barley fed' cattle) or as yellowish areas of necrosis. These are raised slightly above the liver surface, more or less circular in outline and all about 15 mm in diameter. In the early stage the peripheries of the lesions are hyperaemic but at a later stage the necrotic areas become encapsulated.
      Judgement: Reject liver.

(7)   Abscess, e.g. in umbilical pyaemia, which is fairly common in calves. The umbilicus is thickened and full of pus. Abscesses are found in the liver [Plate 3(e)] and kidneys. Petechiae are common in the kidneys. Sepsis occurs in the joints – the so-called 'joint ill'.
      Judgement: Total rejection.
      Liver abscesses are very frequent in 'barley fed' cattle. As these abscesses are often large, they tend to be ruptured during evisceration with resultant contamination of the peritoneum and pleura.
      Judgement: Reject liver. Rejection of the diaphragm and stripping of the peritoneum and pleura may be necessary.

(8)   Tuberculosis (p. 135).

(9)   Actinobacillosis (p. 115).

(10) Cirrhosis – this denotes increase of fibrous connective tissue in the substance of the liver. The commonest cause of this is liver fluke (p. 153).
      Judgement: Reject liver.

(11) *Echinococcus* cysts (p. 148).

(12) *Tenuicollis* cysts (p. 149).

(13) Melanosis (p. 107).

(14) Xanthosis (p. 108).

(15) 'Sawdust liver' or focal necrosis of the liver is a condition of the bovine liver in which there are small areas of necrosis scattered throughout the liver substance. It is caused by bacteria that probably originate in the intestine and travel to the liver by the portal circulation.
      Judgement: Reject liver.

(16) Red-water (p. 158).

Sheep liver

(1)   Hepatitis.
      Judgement: As bovine.

(2)   Peritonitis and cloudy swelling (p. 188).

(3)   Fatty change, e.g. in pregnancy, toxaemia (twin lamb disease).
      Judgement: As bovine.

(4)   Tumours, especially of the lymphatic type (lymphosarcoma p. 193).

(5) *Fasciola hepatica* infection (p. 153).
(6) *Tenuicollis* cysts and tracks (p. 149).
(7) *Echinococcus* cysts (p. 148).
(8) Tyrosine crystals. These occur on the surface of imported frozen canned livers. The contents of the can have a smell of wine, which is due to prolonged storage with consequent breakdown of the liver substance. The crystals appear as white flakes widely scattered over the liver surface and on the inner lining of the opened blood vessels.
   Judgement: total rejection.

Pig liver

(1) Hepatitis.
   Judgement: As bovine.
(2) Peritonitis and cloudy swelling (p. 188).
(3) Fatty change.
   Judgement: As bovine.
(4) Tumours (p. 192).
(5) 'Milk spot' liver (p. 141).
(6) Tuberculosis (p. 135).
(7) *Echinococcus* cysts (p. 148).
(8) *Tenuicollis* cysts (p. 149).
(9) Cirrhosis. this often causes jaundice.
   Judgement: Reject liver or whole carcass and offal when jaundice present.
(10) Hypertrophic cirrhosis. This is associated with regenerative hyperplasia in which liver cells regenerate in an already damaged liver. In this condition the liver is enlarged and cirrhotic. The surface is finely granular like morocco leather, or almost smooth. On section small islets of normal liver tissue are apparent. Pigs with this type of liver are very often jaundiced.
   Judgement: Reject liver. If jaundice is present reject carcass and offal.

Deer liver

(1) Fatty change – especially stag liver during rut.
   Judgement: As bovine.
(2) Enlargement and engorgement with blood – especially stag livers during rut.
   Judgement: Reject liver.
(3) Abscesses (p. 104).
(4) *Tenuicollis* tracts and cysts (p. 149).
(5) Tuberculosis (p. 135).
(6) *Fasciola hepatica* (p. 153).
(7) Contamination and damage due to shooting.
   Judgement: Reject liver.

(8) Listeriosis (p. 129).
(9) *Echinococcus* cysts (p. 148).
(10) Abscess, e.g. in umbilical pyaemia.
   Judgement: As bovine.

Lungs and pleura

Bovine lungs

(1) Pneumonia or inflammation of the lungs. This can be caused by bacteria, viruses, foreign bodies or parasites. There are two main types of pneumonia:

   (a) Broncho-pneumonia, which is characterised by small patches of pneumonia scattered among the normal lung tissue and is an extension of bronchial infection.

   (b) Lobar pneumonia, which is characterised by the involvement of the whole or greater part of a lobe. The hepatised (liver-like) or consolidated tissue is of uniform appearance and separated from the normal lung tissue by a sharp line of demarcation.

   A third type, 'foreign body' pneumonia, can occur due to traumatic injury, e.g. wire puncturing lungs.
   All types of pneumonia can become septic or gangrenous and may spread to the pleura, causing pleurisy.
   Judgement: Total rejection if evidence of system infection, otherwise reject affected parts.

(2) 'Husk' or 'hoose' (p. 144).
(3) Tuberculosis (p. 135).
(4) Interlobular or interstitial emphysema. This is chiefly seen in the lungs of old cows. There is marked dilatation of the interstitial tissue that arises as the result of penetration of air into the interlobular connective tissue accentuating the lobulated appearance of the lung surface [Plate 2(d)].
   Judgement: Reject lungs.

(5) *Echinococcus* cysts (p. 148).
(6) Melanosis (p. 107).
(7) Contamination of trachea and lungs with ingesta and blood. During slaughter, ingesta may be regurgitated from the rumen and aspirated into the trachea and lungs. In such cases the lungs are rejected. In the Jewish and Muslim methods of slaughtering, the trachea may be cut at the same time as the blood vessels of the neck, thus allowing blood to be 'inspired' into the lungs. Such lungs are usually rejected. A somewhat similar condition is seen in the lungs of pigs when water enters the lungs during the scalding process.
   Judgement: Reject lungs.

(8) *Fasciola hepatica* migratory cysts (p. 153).

(9)   Pleurisy (inflammation of the pleura). This is usually associated with a pneumonia and is either acute or chronic. It is important not to confuse acute pleurisy with 'back bleeding' or 'oversticking', which is due to the pleura at the entrance of the chest being punctured during sticking so that blood enters the thorax and congeals on or under the pleura:

    (a)   Tuberculous pleurisy, either acute or chronic ('grapes') (p. 135).

    (b)   Septic pleurisy, which may be the result of a foreign body (e.g. wire). When pus collects in the thorax the condition is known as empyema.

        Judgement: Total rejection if evidence of systemic infection, otherwise reject affected parts.

(10)   Tumours (p. 192).

(11)   Anthracosis. Black or bluish-black pigmentation of lung substance and lymph nodes due to inhalation of coal dust (p. 105).

Sheep lungs

(1)   Lungworm infection, especially *Muellerius capillaris* (p. 145).

(2)   Pneumonia and pleurisy. Acute, chronic or septic. Septic pneumonia is fairly common in sheep. A common cause of pneumonia in sheep is *Pasteurella haemolytica*.

    Judgement: As bovine.

(3)   *Echinococcus* cysts (p. 148).

(4)   Contamination by ingesta and blood as in bovine.

    Judgement: Reject lungs.

(5)   'Blood splashing' – small haemorrhages caused by rise in blood pressure after electrical stunning. (See (2) in next section.)

(6)   *Pulmonary adenomatosis* or *Jaagsiekte* (p. 131).

(7)   Maedi-Visna (p. 129).

Pig lungs

(1)   Enzootic pneumonia (p. 125).

(2)   Blood splashing. This condition is characterised by small capillary haemorrhages throughout the muscles, organs and tissues of the body. It occurs during the slaughtering process no matter what method of slaughter is used, with the exception of the carbon dioxide method of stunning. However, it is certainly much more common when electrical stunning is used.

    When the current is applied the muscles contract strongly, squeezing the blood out of the capillaries. There is also a steep rise in blood pressure. After removal of the electric lethaler the muscles relax. The blood immediately rushes back under high pressure into the empty capillaries. Unless the blood pressure is reduced by 'sticking', many of the capillaries are ruptured. The resulting haemorrhages are known as 'blood splashes'.

To prevent this happening animals should be bled within 5 seconds of stunning. This is not always practicable with many line systems in use at the present time.

Blood splashing occurs in all animals but is commonest in pigs and young lambs electrically stunned. Any organ or tissue can be affected, but it is apparently commonest in those organs in which capillaries are embedded in soft tissue and therefore have little support, e.g. in pig's lungs. Also commonly affected are the pig's diaphragm, abdominal and leg muscles and lamb's mesentery, lungs, diaphragm, neck and abdominal muscles and heart. Lymph nodes of the bovine head and lungs are often affected.

It has been said that 'blood splashed' meat tends to putrefy quickly because of the increased blood content. This is doubtful as is also the statement that proper rest before slaughter reduces the incidence of 'blood splashing'. Dietary factors may play a part.

Judgement: The usual practice is to trim, if localised, and reject the affected parts because the meat is unsaleable. On cooking the haemorrhages become black or dark brown. If circumstances permit the affected parts may be used for manufacturing purposes.

(3)   Pneumonia and pleurisy – commonly in swine fever, swine erysipelas and pig paratyphoid.

Judgement: As bovine.

(4)   Haemorrhages due to invasion by *Ascaris* larvae (p. 141).

(5)   *Echinococcus* cysts (p. 148).

(6)   Tuberculosis (p. 135).

(7)   Tuberculosis of pleura. Occasionally of diffuse type but generally in the form of small discrete nodules that may penetrate through the parietal pleura to the intercostal muscles or the ribs themselves.

Judgement: Reject lungs and undertake all other TB checks.

(8)   Lung worms (p. 145), especially *Metastrongylus apri*. The surface of the affected lungs shows elevated flat areas that have a mother-of-pearl lustre. They are commonest at the extremities of the lungs. Sometimes small nodules may be seen in the lung substance just beneath the pleura. On cutting into the lungs the worms can be found in the bronchioles.

(9)   Back bleeding (p. 195).

Judgement: Reject affected parts.

(10) Glässer's disease adhesions (p. 127).

Deer lungs

(1)   Aspergillosis (p. 166).

(2)   Lung worms (p. 145).

(3)   Pleurisy owing to horn wounds (p. 179).

(4)   Tuberculosis (p. 135).

(5)   *Echinococcus* cysts (p. 148).

Lymph nodes

As has been said in Chapter 6, examination of lymph nodes is of prime importance in meat inspection as they give a guide to the nature and extent of disease
processes in the body. In examination of lymph nodes, it is important to make
deep multiple incisions in the large nodes.If only one or two incisions are made,
small lesions may be missed, e.g. in tuberculosis and actinobacillosis.

Knowledge of a lymph node's drainage area is of importance when rejecting a
lymph node.

Bovine lymph nodes

(1) Tuberculosis (p. 135).
(2) Actinobacillosis (p. 115).
(3) Lymphadenitis (p. 129).
(4) Parasites, e.g. pentastomes (p. 176) and immature flukes (p. 153) in
     mesenteric nodes.
(5) Enzootic leukosis (p. 125).
(6) Anthracosis (p. 105).

Sheep lymph nodes

(1) Lymphadenitis (p. 129).
(2) Parasites (caseous or calcified) (As bovine.)
(3) Caseous lymphadenitis (p. 124).
(4) Lymphosarcoma (p. 193).
(5) Actinobacillosis (p. 115).
(6) Maedi-Visna (p. 129).

Pig lymph nodes

(1) Tuberculosis (p. 135).

  (a) Bovine type. This is very pathogenic for pigs and gives rise to an
       exudative type of reaction in which occur typical tubercles with sub-
       sequent caseation and calcification. Stellate caseation with haemor-
       rhages occurs in virulent infections.
       Judgement: If localised reject local part or organ. Generalised
       tuberculosis or miliary tuberculosis merits total rejection.
  (b) Avian type. This is caused by *Mycobacterium avium* and *M. intra-
       cellularae.* The latter organism has been found in sawdust used for
       bedding. It is not very pathogenic for pigs and gives rise to a
       productive tissue reaction. The nodes are enlarged and firmer than
       normal and at first show no tubercles but later show small yellow foci

or large necrotic areas in the centre of the node. They are putty-like and are readily enucleated. The lesions of avian tuberculosis are generally confined to the lymph nodes of the head and the mesenteric lymph nodes.

Judgement: Reject head and the intestines.

(2)   *Corynebacterium equi.* This causes lesions very similar to tuberculosis in the submaxillary nodes. The lesions are small whitish necrotic foci surrounded by connective tissue capsules and easily enucleated.

Judgement: Reject head.

(3)   Lymphosarcoma (p. 193).
(4)   Lymphadenitis, e.g. swine fever and swine erysipelas (p. 129).
(5)   Abscesses (p. 104).

Judgement: Reject head.

Deer lymph nodes

(1)   Actinobacillosis (p. 115).
(2)   Anthrax (p. 116).
(3)   Jöhne's disease (p. 127).
(4)   Malignant catarrhal fever (p. 130).
(5)   Yersiniosis (p. 139).
(6)   Tuberculosis (p. 135).

Mammary glands

Bovine mammary glands

(1)   Mastitis. This is inflammation of the mammary tissue.

   (a)   Streptococcal mastitis caused by *Streptococcus agalactiae.* This type tends to become chronic. One or more quarters may be affected and the affected areas are indurated.

   Judgement: It is generally only necessary to reject the udder.

   (b)   Septic mastitis and summer mastitis caused by staphylococci or *Corynebacterium pyogenes* may be spread by the sheep head fly *Hydrotaea irritans* (p. 161). The affected areas in the live animal become enlarged, hot and painful. The supramammary lymph nodes become enlarged and oedematous as may also the iliac and sub-lumbar lymph nodes. The udder contains a red or straw-coloured exudate with a putrid odour. Septic areas are present and gangrene may follow.

   Judgement: When there is any evidence of systemic involvement (sepsis) or gangrene develops carcass and offal are rejected.

(2)   Tuberculosis (p. 135).

(3) Tumours (p. 192).
(4) Bruising, especially of the teat (trampling wounds).
    Judgement: Reject affected parts.
(5) Foot and mouth disease (p. 125).
(6) Cowpox. This is a virus disease of cattle generally confined to the teats of cows. The typical lesion is a small vesicle, followed by a scabby sore. It is transmissible to humans.
    Judgement: Local rejection.

Sheep mammary glands

(1) Mastitis, acute or chronic. Septic mastitis is common and this may become gangrenous (p. 112).
(2) Maedi-Visna (p. 129).
    Judgement: Depending upon seriousness of the condition it may be necessary only to reject the udder. If, however, there is sepsis or gangrene present the carcass and offal are rejected.

Pig mammary glands

(1) Mastitis (p. 183).
(2) Actinomycosis (p. 116).
(3) Tuberculosis (p. 135).
(4) Abscesses (p. 104).
(5) Melanosis ('seedy cut' or 'seedy belly') (p. 107).
    Judgement: If there are no further complications, in all of these five types of udder condition only the udder is rejected.

Muscle

Bovine muscle

(1) Bruises (p. 100), haematomata (p. 101) and abscesses (p. 104).
    Judgement: Reject affected parts.
(2) *Cysticercus bovis* (masseter muscles) (p. 152).
(3) Interstitial myositis or steatosis [Plate 4(a)] or muscular fibrosis, or lipomatosis of muscles. There is progressive replacement of muscle tissue by adipose tissue without alteration in gross form of the muscle.
    Judgement: Reject affected parts.
(4) Actinobacillosis (masseter muscles most commonly affected) (p. 115).
(5) Sarcocysts (p. 157).
(6) Blood splashing (p. 180).
(7) Eosinophilic myositis (p. 106).

(8)   Blackquarter (p. 118).

(9)   Xanthosis (p. 108).

(10) Nodular necrosis or Roekl's granuloma. This generally occurs in old cows as greyish yellow nodules up to the size of a golf ball in the muscle tissue. It is commonest in the muscles of the tail.

>   *Judgement:* Reject affected parts.

(11) Bone taint (p. 103).

Sheep muscle

(1)   Bruises (p. 100), haematomata (p. 101) and abscesses (p. 104).

>   *Judgement:* Reject affected parts.

(2)   *Cysticercus ovis* (p. 150).

(3)   Sarcocysts (p. 157).

(4)   Blood splashing (p. 180).

(5)   Steatosis (p. 184).

(6)   Injection abscesses in neck and shoulder muscles.

>   *Judgement:* Trim.

(7)   Blackquarter (p. 118).

>   *Judgement:* Total rejection.

Pig muscle

(1)   Bruises (p. 100), haematomata (p. 101) and abscesses (p. 104).

>   *Judgement:* Reject affected parts.

(2)   Sarcocysts (p. 157)

(3)   *Cysticercus cellulosae* (p. 152).

(4)   Blood splashing (p. 180).

(5)   Pale soft exudate (p. 108).

(6)   *Echinococcus* cysts (especially in sows).

(7)   Dark firm and dry (p. 106).

(8)   Sexual odour (p. 102).

Deer muscle

(1)   Shooting injuries.

>   *Judgement:* Reject damaged and contaminated parts.

(2)   Blackquarter (p. 118).

(3)   Warbles (p. 158).

(4)   Avian tuberculosis (p. 139).

(5)   Sexual odour (p. 102).

Skin

Pig skin

The skin of the pig is most commonly affected. Conditions found are:

(1) Acute congestion or inflammation in such conditions as acute swine fever (p. 134) and erysipelas (p. 133).

(2) Urticaria as in swine erysipelas ('diamonds') and pig paratyphoid (p. 131). [Plate 5(c)].

(3) Transit erythema or 'lime burning'. This usually affects pigs travelling long journeys, and tends to take the form of a red rash or red patches on the skin of the belly and hams, i.e. those parts that come into contact with floors of vehicles. It is caused by the irritant effect of urine or disinfectant and the constant rubbing or friction. The condition varies from very slight to very severe. Where the irritation is severe, the subcutaneous fat becomes red and the adjacent lymph nodes are congested.
   Judgement: Trim and reject affected parts.

(4) Bruising. Two common causes of this are (i) 'stick' marks due to hitting with sticks; (ii) teeth marks due to fighting. These are generally typical marks, the stick mark being two straight red weals with a clear area in between them, whereas teeth marks are generally irregularly shaped and curved red marks on the skin. If the bruising is severe, a haematoma may be formed., i.e. when haemorrhage takes place either in the form of clotted or unclotted blood under the unbroken skin.
   Judgement: Reject affected parts.

(5) Abscesses (often due to infected bites) (p. 104).

(6) Shotty eruption or sooty mange. This consists of numerous papules, black in colour, in which curled, elongted hairs, and a black sebaceous material are found. It is said to be caused by a coccidium, but this is doubtful. It is commonest on the skin of the buttocks.
   Judgement: Reject affected parts of skin.

(7) Mange (p. 162).

(8) Ringworm (trichophytosis) (p. 166).

(9) Pityriasis rosea. This is a disease generally of young pigs, and resembles ringworm. It begins as small red papules on the skin of abdomen and inner thighs. The papules expand centrifugally to produce at first scaly plaques and later, when the central areas return to normal, ring-shaped lesions that are red and scaly. As the rings expand gthey coalesce to produce mosaic patterns. The cause is unknown, but there is strong evidence that it is congenital in origin.
   Judgement: Reject affected parts of skin.

(10) Damage to extremities, e.g. tips of ears, tail and feet: haematoma (p. 101) of the ear is common when the ear flap is swollen and ballooned and full of

blood. Necrotic tails and abscessed tails due to biting are fairly common [Plate 4(c)]. It is always advisable, when tails are damaged, to have the carcasss split, as abscesses are often found in the pelvic region and spinal column (p. 104).

(11)   Foot and mouth disease lesions (p. 125).
(12)   Swine vesicular disease lesions (p. 135).

Bovine skin

This is not so liable to damage and infection as the pig's skin because of the hair covering. The conditions that may be seen as well as bruises, etc. are:

(1)   Ringworm (p. 166): trichophytosis (*T. verrucosum*).
(2)   Foot and mouth disease lesions (p. 125).
(3)   Tumours, especially papillomata (warts) (p. 192).
(4)   'Foul of the foot'. This is a condition in which infection gains entrance to foot and lower joints with the formation of pus, necrosis of tissues, and swelling of the foot and joints. It is caused by *Bacteroides necrophorus*.
        Judgement: Reject affected parts.
(5)   'Skin tuberculosis'. These are nodules in the subcutaneous layers of the skin up to the size of a hen's egg and very similar to tuberculous lesions in appearance. They are commonest in the legs and shoulder region. It is an important condition in the live animal as the animal so affected can react to the tuberculin test. It is very unusual for the regional lymph nodes to be involved. Very similar lesions are caused by Jöhne's disease vaccine.
        Judgement: Local trimming.
(6)   Warble fly larvae – the so-called 'licked back' and warble holes in the skin (p. 158).
(7)   Mucosal disease (p. 130).
(8)   Listeriosis (p. 129).
(9)   Lice (p. 162).

Sheep skin

(1)   Sheep scab (p. 163).
(2)   Fly strike (p. 161).
(3)   Foot and mouth disease lesions (p. 125).
(4)   Foot rot. This is a common condition in sheep causing lameness. It is caused by a mixed infection of *bacteroides nodosus* and *Bacteroides necrophorus*.
        Judgement: Reject feet.
(5)   Orf (see p. 130).
(6)   Ringworm, especially of the skin of the head, caused by *Trichophyton verrucosum*.

(7) Lice (p. 162).
(8) *Ixodes ricinus* (p. 164).
(9) Scrapie (p. 133).
(10) Ringworm (p. 166).

Deer skin

(1) Actinomycosis (p. 116).
(2) Deer ked (p. 160).
(3) *Ixodes ricinus* (p. 164).
(4) *Hydrotaea irritans* (p. 161).
(5) Papillomata (p. 192).
(6) Horn wounds.
(7) Warble fly larvae (p. 158).
(8) Lice (p. 162).
(9) Bites in muntjac bucks during rutting season, on hindquarters. The buck has protruding lower canine teeth that are very sharp.

Spleen

Bovine spleen

(1) Tuberculosis – substance in congenital tuberculosis, capsule other types (p. 135).
(2) Anthrax (p. 116).
(3) Red-water (p. 158).
(4) Chronic venous congestion (so-called slaughter spleen).
(5) Leukaemia – spleen enlarged (p. 168).
(6) Infarcts (p. 174).
(7) *Echinococcus* cysts. These tend to become very big in the spleen (p. 148).
(8) Haematoma (traumatic in origin) (p. 101).
(9) Peritonitis (inflammation of the peritoneum) – characterised by the peritoneum adhering to the surface of the abdominal cavity or the organs within the abdominal cavity such as the spleen, liver, stomach and intestines. Can often become septic.
    Judgement: Total rejection if evidence of systemic infection, otherwise reject affected parts.

Sheep spleen

The sheep spleen is not often found to be affected by diseased conditions but the following can occur:

(1) Peritonitis (p. 188).
(2) Leukaemia (p. 168).
(3) *Echinococcus* cysts (p. 148).
(4) *Tenuicollis* cysts (p. 149).

Pig spleen

(1) Chronic venous congestion due to torsion. This occurs because the spleen is very loosely attached to the stomach by the omentum. The congestion occurs becauser the veins, being thinner walled than the arteries, are more constricted by the torsion.
(2) Chronic enlargement – swine erysipelas (p. 133).
(3) Tuberculosis (especially miliary) (p. 135).
(4) Haematoma (p. 101).
(5) Anthrax (p. 116).
(6) Leukaemia (p. 168).
(7) *Echinococcus* cysts (p. 148).
    Judgement: Reject spleen.

Deer spleen

(1) Tuberculosis (p. 135).
(2) Contamination (p. 6).
(3) Anthrax (p. 116).

Stomach and intestines

Bovine stomach and intestine

(1) Peptic ulcers in the abomasum of the calf.
    Judgement: Reject affected parts.
(2) Actinobacillosis of reticulum and rumen (p. 115).
(3) Enteritis (p. 124).
(4) Peritonitis (p. 188).
(5) Pimply gut (p. 142).
(6) Jöhne's disease (p. 127).
(7) Tuberculosis of the mesenteric lymph nodes and the intestine (p. 135).
(8) Pentastome larvae in the mesenteric lymph nodes (p. 176).
(9) Traumatic reticulitis. This results from perforation due to a foreign body, e.g. nail, fence wire or baling wire. A peritonitis develops, with or without abscess formation. This may become walled off by fibrous tissue. Complications may follow, e.g. traumatic pericarditis, septic pleurisy, pneumonia, diaphragmatic hernia and liver abscesses.

Judgement: Local trimming may suffice but severe cases can lead to the rejection of the carcass and offal.

Sheep stomach and intestine

(1) Parasitic gastritis and enteritis (p. 124).
(2) Jöhne's disease (p. 127).
(3) Caseous and calcified parasitic lesions in the mesenteric lymph nodes.

Pig stomach and intestine

(1)   Enteritis (p. 124).
(2)   Peritonitis (p. 188).
(3)   Tuberculosis of the mesenteric lymph nodes (p. 135).
(4)   *Ascaris suum* infection (p. 141).
(5)   *Hyostrongylus rubidus* infection (p. 142).
(6)   Swine fever (p. 134).
(7)   Pig paratyphoid (p. 131).
(8)   Oedema of the stomach wall in bowel oedema.
        Judgement: Reject stomach and identify cause.
(9)   Anthrax (p. 116).
(10) Mesenteric or intestinal emphysema. This is a rare condition that affects pigs. Small, spherical bubbles occur in grape-like clusters in the mesenteric lymph vessels close to the intestine. They measure up to 10 mm in diameter and the majority are clear although some are blood stained. When pressed they burst easily with a popping noise. The cause is unknown.
        Judgement: Reject mesentery and intestines.

Deer stomach and intestine

(1) Tuberculosis (p. 135).
(2) Yersiniosis (p. 139).
(3) Jöhne's disease (p. 127).
(4) Malignant catarrhal fever (p. 130).
(5) Abomasal and intestinal ulceration. This condition is often associated with winter death syndrome and other stress conditions. There are ulcers in the abomasum and intestines, perforation of which leads to peritonitis.
        Judgement: Total rejection if evidence of systemic infections such as septicaemia, pyaemia and toxaemia or emaciation found, otherwise reject affected parts.
(6) Parasites (p. 140).

Uterus

Bovine uterus

(1) Metritis or inflammation of the uterus:

    (a) Septic metritis is a serious condition and carcasses are usually rejected.
        Judgement: total rejection.

    (b) Chronic endometritis – characterised by a mucopurulent discharge without fever and is regarded as a local condition.
        Judgement: Reject genital tract.

    (c) Pyometra – pus in the uterus. Seen in 'white heifer disease', which is a condition in white heifers with imperforate hymen with consequent retention of the uterine secretions.
        Judgement: Reject genital tract.

(2) Mummified fetus. The dead fetus becomes dehydrated. It is aseptic and odourless.
    Judgement: Reject genital tract.

(3) Tuberculous metritis either as a result of haematogenous spread or as a descending infection spread from peritoneum via the fallopian tubes to the uterus.
    Judgement: Dependent upon how widespread the condition is throughout the other organs and carcass.

(4) Tumours (p. 192).

(5) Retained fetal membranes.
    Judgement: Reject genital tract, but if the carcass has an abnormal odour total rejection is necessary.

(6) Brucellosis (p. 123).

Sheep uterus

(1) Metritis
    Judgement: As bovine.

(2) Pregnancy toxaemia or 'twin lamb disease'. This is a condition that develops in ewes about 14 days before lambing and is more common during severe weather. There is generally a fatty liver.
    Judgement: Reject liver. The carcass is judged on its merits.

(3) Tumours (p. 192).

(4) Mummified fetus.
    Judgement: Reject uterus.

Pig uterus

(1) Metritis (see above).
    Judgement: As for bovine.

(2)   Mummified and macerated fetuses.
      Judgement: Reject uterus.
(3)   Tumours (see below).

Tumours

Tumours are abnormal growths of new tissue arising by unknown cause from pre-existing body cells, having no purposeful function and being characterised by a tendency to autonomous and unrestrained growth. In some instances the tumour cells are normal in appearance, faithful reproductions of their parent types; such tumours are generally benign. Other tumours are composed of cells slightly different from normal adult types, different in appearance, size, shape and structure; these tumours are usually malignant. Thus we have two main types of tumour: (1) benign and (2) malignant (cancer).

Benign tumours

These consist of cells showing no great variation from those of normal tissue and most are encapsulated and tend to remain localised. They are frequently multiple, several arising in different parts of the body either simultaneously or in succession. In such cases all the tumours are identical. Examples of benign tumours are:

(1)   Lipoma – a tumour of fat cells
(2)   Fibroma – a tumour of fibrous tissue cells
(3)   Chondroma – a tumour of cartilaginous cells
(4)   Osteoma – a tumour of bone cells
(5)   Papilloma (wart) – a tumour of skin cells
(6)   Adenoma – a tumour of glandular cells.
      Judgement: Affected parts are rejected.

Malignant tumours (cancer)

These consist of abnormal tissue cells and are not capsulated. They have tremendous growth energy and largely lack the growth restraint that characterises normal tissue. The cells may invade normal and adjacent tissues by direct or continuous growth or may infiltrate within blood and lymph vessels where they are broken off and carried to distant organs in which they lodge through filtration, a process known as metastasis. The ability of those cells to grow when deposited elsewhere is a characteristic feature of malignant tumours. The simplest classification of malignant tumours is into two types: (1) carcinoma and (2) sarcoma.
    There are many types of these, depending on the tissue cells from which they

arise. Carcinoma spreads throughout the body by way of the lymph stream and sacroma by the bloodstream, except in the case of the melanotic variety and lymphosarcoma. Carcinoma is generally a disease of middle or old age, whereas sarcoma can occur at any age.

As most food animals are slaughtered early in life, the commonest type of cancer found is sarcoma, e.g. lymphosarcoma. Carcinomas are generally found in old cows.

Metastases are usually found in liver, lungs, spleen, kidneys and lymph nodes.

Melanomas are common in old grey horses, particularly in the skin of the tail and perineal region. They are generally benign but occasionally malignant with metastases in the lungs, liver and spleen. Plate 4(d) shows a pig skin melanoma.

In cattle, tumorous changes (other than haemangiomas, or papillomas or warts) are notifiable.

Judgement: This depends upon size and number of the tumours. Organs affected are rejected, but in the case of the carcass, local trimming may be all that is necessary. Carcasses affected with multiple tumours are rejected.

Hypertrophy

A condition in which the cells of a tissue or organ increase in size and number. It can occur either:

(1) physiologically, e.g. mammary glands in pregnancy and lactation.
      Judgement: Fit.
(2) Pathologically, or as it is known, compensatory hypertrophy. This is best seen when one kidney is deficient – the other kidney takes over the function of the deficient one and becomes very much enlarged.
      Judgement: Fit for human consumption.

Muscular hypertrophy or double muscling

This condition occurs in cattle and occasionally in sheep. The increase in size of the muscles is due to a greater number of muscle cells and not to 'double muscles', which is a misnomer. The enlargement may affect all muscles but most often the neck, shoulders and muscles of the upper hind limbs. The condition is hereditary and affects many breeds of cattle. As well as an increase in muscle of up to about 20%, there is a decrease in subcutaneous muscle and carcass fat, with the result that the muscles are clearly demarcated from each other. The internal organs, e.g. the heart, liver, spleen and kidneys, are greatly reduced in size. Obviously the increase in muscle and decrease in fat are advantages, but there are certain disadvantages as the live animals are more liable to bruising and fractures, stress and difficult calving because of the large size of the calves. There is also a decrease in the amount of edible offal.

Atrophy

Wasting of tissue which may occur in any tissue. This also can occur:

(1)   Physiologically, e.g. atrophy of the thymus or atrophy of muscles through lack of use.
        Judgement: Fit.
(2)   Pathologically – generally associated with old age or low intake of food. Pressure atrophy is commonly seen in meat inspection, e.g. hydronephrosis when kidney cells are atrophied owing to back pressure of urine and in gid when there is pressure atrophy of brain and even skull bones.
        Judgement: Reject affected parts.

Fat necrosis

This occurs as white, opaque areas of fat scattered throughout the normal fat. It is most often found in the abdominal cavity, particularly in the kidney fat of pig and ox. The probable cause is leakage of pancreatic juice from the pancreas, which contains the enzymes lipase and trypsin. These act upon the fat and produce the typical lesions [Plate 6(e)].

When fat necrosis occurs outside the abdominal cavity, it may be due to abnormal conditions of the pancreas, e.g. acute pancreatitis, or to injury to fatty tissue – traumatic fat necrosis. A common example of this is fat necrosis of the brisket in cattle – the so-called 'putty brisket' or presternal calcification.

Another type of fat necrosis occurs mainly in Channel Islands cattle. This is a widespread necrosis of the abdominal fat, the cause of which is unknown. Large firm masses of necrotic fat are formed, which on the cut surface are firm, generally dry and yellow. When these masses form around the intestine, ureters or kidneys, constriction of these occur and the result may be fatal.

Judgement: Dependent upon the degree of affection, but local trimming is generally all that is necessary.

Butchers' Joints and Meat Products

Chapter 18
Butchers' Joints

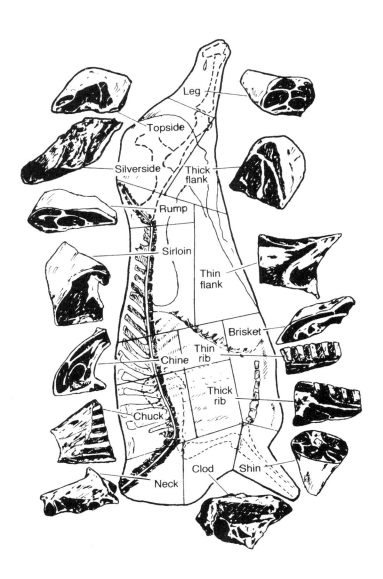

Fig. 18.1   Joints of beef.

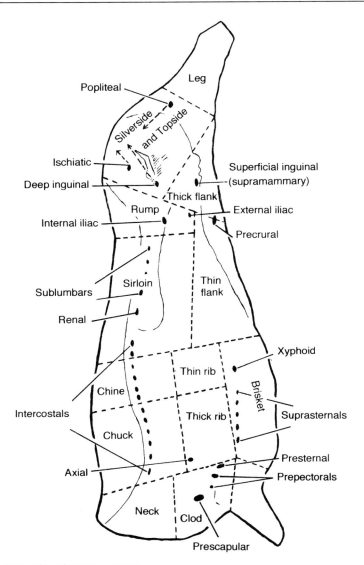

Fig. 18.2   Joints of beef with lymph nodes.

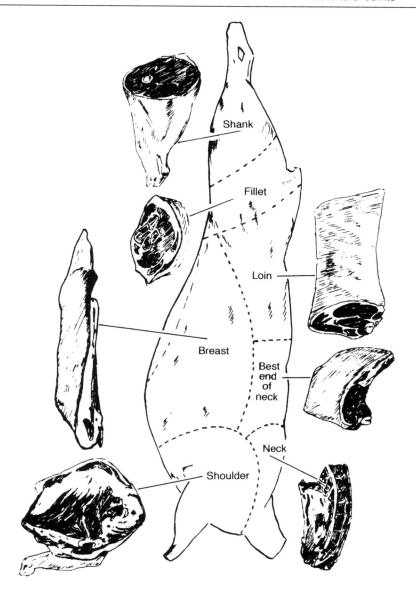

Fig. 18.3   Joints of lamb.

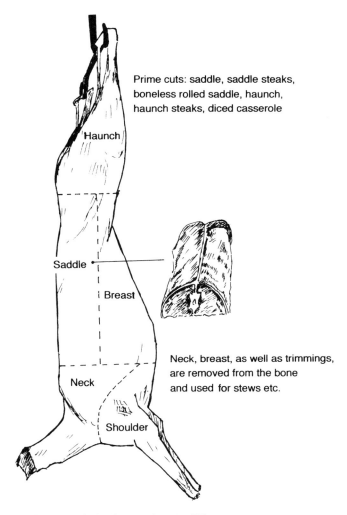

Prime cuts: saddle, saddle steaks,
boneless rolled saddle, haunch,
haunch steaks, diced casserole

Haunch

Saddle

Breast

Neck, breast, as well as trimmings,
are removed from the bone
and used for stews etc.

Neck

Shoulder

Fig. 18.4   Joints of venison. (**NB**   Carcass is not split.)

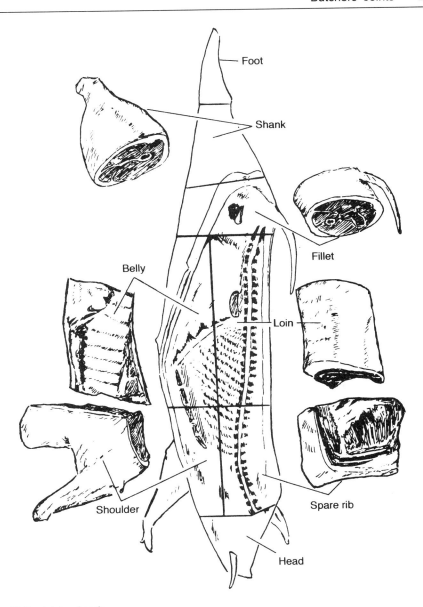

Fig. 18.5 Joints of pork.

Chapter 19

Meat Preservation and Meat Products

Unless meat is preserved in some way it soon putrefies. This is due to the action of bacteria, moulds and yeasts. These obtain nourishment from the meat and in so doing alter it in various ways. To grow and proliferate the organisms need temperatures favourable to them. It is therefore customary to classify organisms as follows:

(1) *Psychrophiles*, which have an optimum temperature range of –2 to 7°C.
(2) *Mesophiles*, which have an optimum temperature range of 10 to 40°C.
(3) *Thermophiles*, which have an optimum temperature range of 43 to 66°C.

It is thus possible to preserve meat by subjecting it to temperatures approximating to:

(1) –2°C (sub-optimal temperatures) by chilling or freezing.
(2) 66°C (super-optimal temperatures) by pasteurising, cooking or sterilising.

Organisms also need water for growth and so it is possible to preserve meat by removing this by dehydration, freezing or curing.

Some bacteria, e.g. *Clostridium perfringens*, liquefy the connective tissue in meat, causing it to disintegrate. Gases such as hydrogen sulphide, carbon dioxide, ammonia and indole are produced. The glycogen or muscle sugar is fermented giving rise to acetic or butyric acids, which cause offensive smells and tastes.

Discoloration is caused by changes in the myoglobin or muscle pigment. Brown, green and yellow colours appear when the myoglobin is acted upon by oxygen, hydrogen sulphide and hydrogen peroxide, which are produced by the bacteria present. Discoloration may also be due to pigments produced by various organisms, e.g. *Pseudomonas, Serratia marcescens*, Micrococci and yeasts give rise to greens, reds and pinks. Moulds also produce pigments, e.g. *Cladosporium, Sporotrichum* and *Penicillium* give black, white and bluish green, respectively.

Preservation by cold

Meats can be preserved by chilling and freezing. This is the simplest and easiest method of preservation and is the basis of refrigeration. By refrigeration, meat can be kept for long periods with relatively little deterioration in appearance, texture and flavour.

In 1842, H. Benjamin in England was granted a patent for freezing foods by immersing them in an ice and salt brine.

Preservationi by cold or refrigeration depends on the fact that bacteria are unable to multiply at low temperatures, mainly due to the fact that water, which is necessary for this, is changed to ice. Another factor is that most of the harmful bacteria grow best at body temperature (37°C). It is very important to remember that bacteria are resistant to cold but are not killed by it. Live bacteria have been found in ice core samples that came from over 140 metres deep in the Antarctic. The bacteria may be at least 10 000 years old. When the temperature rises and the meat thaws out, the bacteria start to multiply and may cause the formation of 'surface slime'. Three conditions are necessary for this formation: (1) contamination, (2) temperature at which bacteria can grow, i.e. above freezing, and (3) moisture, which allows the contamination to spread, e.g. sweating on chilled and frozen beef. It is formed by the growth of aerobic spoilage bacteria, such as *Achromobacter* (commonest on beef), *Pseudomonas*, *Streptococcus*, *Proteus*, *Lactobacillus* and *Micrococcus* (commonest on pork). These bacteria grow in colonies that eventually coalesce to form confluent areas of slime. The further apart the individual colonies are originally, i.e. the lower the initial contamination, the longer it will take the slime to form. The bacteria break down the meat giving rise to sour and foul odours. Later the slime may become pigmented owing to contamination by yeasts and moulds. Slime formation on sausages may be entirely due to yeasts.

When slime becomes evident it has been estimated that there are more than 50 000 000 bacteria per square centimetre of surface.

Chilling of meat

This method is useful when meat has to be preserved for a relatively short time, up to 35 days. Chilled meat loses very little in appearance, nutritive value and taste. It is kept at between −1.4°C (meat freezes at −1.4°C) and 1°C, preferably in the dark as light has the effect of oxidising fats. Light liberates free fatty acids and the fat becomes rancid. The atmosphere should be kept dry to prevent mould formation, for which moisture is necessary. A concentration of 5–10% carbon dioxide helps to prevent the growth of moulds and bacteria.

After slaughter most carcasses are chilled in chill rooms in which cold air is circulated bringing the temperature down to −1°C. It is important that the temperature does not reach −1.4°C otherwise the meat will freeze.

If the chilling process is too rapid, cold shortening occurs, which is an undesirable feature.

Cold shortening
Toughness develops in lamb carcasses, particularly if they are exposed to low temperatures within about 16 hours after slaughter. This is due to cold shortening of the muscles. While the pH is about 6.3 and the ATP levels are high, lowering of the temperature causes the muscles to contract. It normally starts at 15°C and becomes greater down to 0°C. This causes toughness of meat on cooking. Beef carcasses do not chll as quickly as lamb carcasses because of the thickness of the muscles. However, the superficial layers may be affected.

Cold shortening is not a problem in pig carcasses because the pH falls more rapidly than in the other animals. Also the pigs' skins and the subcutaneous fat protect the underlying muscles from the rapid cooling. Therefore, pig carcasses can be cooled more rapidly.

Good chilling practices are probably the most important factors in the keeping quality of meat:

(1)   Carcasses should not touch each other.
(2)   Hot carcasses should not be mixed with cold carcasses.
(3)   Chill-room doors should be kept closed as much as possible.
(4)   Chill-room should not be overloaded.
(5)   Chill-room temperature should be checked regularly.
(6)   Avoid excessive condensation to prevent frost forming on chill-room equipment.

Chilled carcasses require an adequate supply of air around them and so have to be hung on hooks, which is rather space consuming. Frozen carcasses, however, can be stacked and therefore require less space.

Freezing of meat

Temperatures in ordinary freezing vary between –18 and –5°C. Frozen meat can be kept for a long time. Frozen beef has a storage life of about 12 months, veal slightly less, mutton and lamb about 8 months and pork about 6 months without too much deterioration. Frozen meat stored too long becomes dry, less palatable and rancid. After thawing it is less durable than fresh-killed or chilled meat.

When frozen meat is thawed it weeps or drips. A watery blood-stained fluid called *drip* escapes. This consists mainly of water, salt, extractives, protein and damaged blood corpuscles. Weeping or drip is an undesirable feature and is caused mainly by the rupture of the muscle cells by large crystals of ice. The loss of weight due to drip in beef is up to 3%. The loss is greater in beef than in mutton, lamb or pork.

Freezing of meat constitutes a change of state because an irreversible change takes place in the sarcoplasm or muscle protein at –2°C (remember that meat freezes at –1.4°C).

Muscle and fat are poor conductors of heat and during slow freezing a large proportion of the fluid in the muscle cells passes through the cell walls and collects between the muscle fibres. There it freezes into ice crystals. The slower the freezing process the larger the ice crystals becoming and because of their size more damage is one to the meat. On thawing, these extracellular ice crystals produce fluid, some of which is not reabsorbed. This produces drip. If, however, freezing takes place very quickly, the ice crystals are very small and are formed within the cells. Less damage is done to the meat and on thawing less drip is produced. One method of quicker freezing is called *blast freezing*, in which cold air is blown on to the meat. The ice crystals reach their maximum size between –1 and –4°C, called the 'zone of maximum ice crystal formation'. After initial freezing it is therefore important to store meat below –4°C. The extent of drip is determined by various factors:

(1) Amount of damage caused to the muscles by freezing and cold storing.
(2) Size and shape of meat. This includes ratio of cut surface to volume and directions of cuts in relation to the axis of the muscle fibres. These factors are more important in beef than in mutton or pork as more cutting is required to produce the right size.

If muscle is frozen before rigor mortis sets in, there is marked contraction on thawing ('thaw rigor') and excessive drip unless the muscle is held taut, e.g. as in a whole carcass of lamb. This is important because of the newer methods of freezing lamb carcasses. These are blast-frozen straught from the slaughter line, when warm and before rigor mortis occurs.

Australian beef quarters are chilled for 3 days at about 1°C and then frozen for 5 days at –10°C. However, in the new processes, with smaller cuts than quarters, increased rates of freezing are used. The hot meat immediately after slaughter is put into a blast tunnel freezer at –35 to –40°C without any previous chilling.

Table 19.1 lists the visual characteristics of beef. Frozen mutton and lamb can be recognised by the flattened cod fat and grey colour of the surface as opposed

Table 19.1 Characteristics of beef

Type	Surface	Flesh	Fat
Home killed	Cold and dry. Sheen on fascia	Bright red colour	Yellow or white and shiny. Tends to be lobulated
Chilled	Cold, damp, sweaty and dull	Pinky red or slatey blue	Pinkish white. Tends to be lobulated
Frozen	Cold, moist, no sheen – drips when thawing	Pale red	Dull white. Flattened

to the light sheen of the home killed. Frozen pork has a darker skin than home killed pork, the muscle is paler and the fat harder.

Freezer burn

This is the name given to yellowish brown or whitish areas seen on the surface of frozen meats. It is due to excessive drying of the surface and can be caused when unprotected meat is blast-frozen or when meat comes into close contact with refrigeration pipes or is placed too close to cold air inlets. The phenomenon involves the formation of a condensed layer of muscular tissue just under the surface. This prevents moisture coming to the surface from the depth of the meat. Excessive surface drying then follows.

   Judgement: Local trimming is all that is necessary.

Preservation by heat

In 1809, Appert, a Frenchman, devised a method of preserving food by heating and bottling. A year later in 1810, Peter Durand, an Englishman, conceived and patented the idea of using tin cans instead of bottles.

   The keeping qualities of canned and bottled goods depend to a large extent upon the sterilisation of the contents. This sterilisation does not bear the full sense of the term used by the bacteriologist, but it does achieve the destruction of food spoilage organisms and is known as 'commercial sterility'.

The canning of corned beef

The cans in the nineteenth century were made of heavy tin plate and were filled through a hole in one end over which a tinned iron disc was soldered. These have now been replaced by the sanitary can in which the end is seamed on.

   Nowadays the cans are made from tinplate. The tin is usually deposited electrically, this having the advantage over hot dipping in that the layer of tin is more uniform. Sometimes the cans are lacquered either before or after forming.

   The body blank of the can is cut out automatically and the body is joined by a double seam, which is hammered and then soldered. The ends are rolled on after suitable rubber or plastic gaskets have been fitted.

Raw material

Meat for corned beef should be of good quality. Freshly killed meat may be used but it is usual to use well chilled beef carcasses trimmed free of cartilage, tendons, connective tissue, excess fat, bruises, blood clots and skin.

Preparation

The boned and trimmed meat selected for canning is cut into approximately 5-cm strips by hand or, preferably, by means of a rotary disc cutter. If the meat is to be cut by hand it is advisable to have a refrigerated cutting room. Meat cutters of the grinder type when fitted with 2.5-or 4-cm plates and a two-blade knife may be used. However, the finished product does not have the attractive appearance of that cut by hand or by a rotary disc cutter.

The general practice is to weigh the meat in suitable size batches and then to put it through the cutter or mincer, and deliver it directly into perforated steel baskets.

Pre-cooking

The perforated baskets are then lowered into the cooking kettles. These are usually made of mild steel and the water in them is heated by steam injection. After the meat has been cooked in the boiling water for 20 minutes, the baskets are drained and the meat is tipped on to stainless steel tables for inspection and further trimming. The trimmings are put through a fine mincer and are added back at a later stage.

After inspection the meat is put into a mixer. Salt at the rate of 1.5% of the original weight of meat and sodium nitrite at the rate of 6 g per 50 kg original weight are dissolved in water and added. About 2 litres of water per 50 kg meat are used.

The yield of cured meat is about 60% of the original weight of the fresh-trimmed meat. The mixed contents are then taken to the filling section.

Filling

The cans are filled by rotary stuffers. The approximate weight of meat required to fill the can is put into the pocket of the stuffer and during rotation a plunger forces the meat into the can. This method of filling is essential with hole and cap tins, but with the modern round or rectangular straight-sided cans filling can be done by hand. After the can is filled it is check weighed and adjusted where necessary.

Closing

This is normally done with mechanical vacuum seamers.

Can washing

The cans are washed immediately after closing so that only clean cans go into the retorts.

Inspection

With rectangular cans, inspection is carried out immediately after washing so as to ensure that the sides of the cans are adequately collapsed, thus indicating that vacuum closing has been properly done.

Processing

The cans are heated in retorts under strict time and temperature controls:

(1)   198 g (7 oz) cans: 55 minutes at 115°C (240°F)
(2)   340 g (12 oz): 80 minutes at 115°C (240°F)
(3)   2.7 kg (6 lb): 4 hours at 115°C (240°F).

Final cooling

After processing, rapid cooling of the cans is essential if overcooking is to be prevented. Unless care is taken, distortion of the can may result. The modern method is to blow the steam out of the retorts with compressed air and then to fill the retorts with water while the pressure is maintained. Sufficient heat must be retained by the cans to ensure rapid drying and so prevent rusting. The water used for cooling must be of potable quality as a safeguard against contamination of contents through leaking seams.

The Aberdeen outbreak of typhoid in 1965 was caused by contamination of the contents of an Argentinian can of corned beef that was cooled by unchlorinated river water.

After cans have been cooled, they are passed through a detergent bath to facilitate handling, lacquering and labelling.

Incubation

The cans are now incubated at 40°C for 1 week or 25°C for 2 weeks. This procedure is based on the fact that most contaminating bacteria that may get into cans will multiply and will make their presence obvious by producing gas and causing blown cans. Inspection of the cans is carried out at specified intervals during the incubation periods. Should the rejection rate be above average, the whole batch may be rejected.

Meat extract

The canning of corned beef is normally accompanied by the production of meat extract. The water in which meat is pre-cooked extracts creatinine and other soluble products from the meat. It is usual to obtain meat extract at the rate of about 2% of the weight of raw meat used. This by-product is an extremely valuable one.

Spoilage of canned goods

Spoilage can occur when the contents have not been sufficiently prepared so that some of the original bacterial flora remains as well as contaiminating bacteria and moulds.

Some canned goods are prepared in such a way that sterility is not possible, e.g. canned pasteurised hams. After pre-cooking the hams at 70–80°C for 8–12 hours the canning is usually carried out at 70°C in open kettles or vessels. The salt and other chemicals present in those products usually prevent the germination and growth of spores.

The common canned ham spoilage is souring ('flat sours') caused by excessive contamination by *Streptococcus faecalis* and lactobacilli, and inadequate heat treatment in cooking or canning. The reduced bacterial contamination should be kept at a low level by continuous refrigeration at 1–2°C between manufacturing and retailing. This is not always practicable and so there is quite a lot of spoilage in this commodity.

Inspection of canned goods

Spoilage in canned goods generally refers to changes in the cans which can be recognised by normal inspection technique. This entails physical examination of the exterior, noting the general condition of the can and its label, e.g. rust, leaks (especially at seams), dents, perforations, stains and visible bulging. Palpation is important in judging the resistance to finger pressure. Some people place great reliance on the percussion note when the can is struck. A dull note denotes soundness, a resonant note unsoundness. When appeal to the contents is necessary, the examination is of two types:

(1) Physical condition – pressure escape of gas or contents on opening, amount of head space, colour, consistency, smell and taste and the colour of the inner surface of the can.
(2) Chemical and bacteriological conditions, which may only be determined by laboratory techniques.

Gas production occurs in most forms of bacterial spoilage. This is indicated by successive changes in the end contour of cans:

(1) '*Flipper*' __ one end of the can bulges when the opposite end is struck.
(2) '*Springer*' – one end is bulged and when this is pressed the other end springs out.
(3) '*Soft blown*' – when thumb pressure momentarily allows reduction.
(4) '*Blown*' or '*Swell*' – when both ends are bulging and neither is reducible.

'Sulphiding' is a term used to indicate black staining of the inside of the can and contiguous parts of the contents. It is caused by the sulphur content of protein foods reacting with unlacquered tin plate. It is only of importance because it is unsightly and can be ignored apart from trimming.

Although all abnormal cans are regarded as unfit, a problem does arise when the cans are only dented and the contents are sound.

If it is obvious that the abnormality is caused by the damage, e.g. if the can is dented and one end is slightly bulged, it could be assumed that the contents will be sound.

Every case must be judged on its merits and every care must be taken and no risks run. There can be an outlet for such goods and that is where cans may be opened under expert supervision and any doubtful cans rejected.

To sum up – the appearance of a good canned commodity requires that:

(1)   The can should be bright and clean.
(2)   There is no rust.
(3)   There are no perforations – physical or corrosive.
(4)   The seams are sound.
(5)   The ends are flat or concave.
(6)   The contents of a solid pack are solid. Sometimes solid packs, unless kept cool, will give a sloppy sound when shaken.
(7)   There should be no evidence of re-sealing.

Upon opening:

(8)   There should be a breaking of the vacuum and not a release of gas or contents.
(9)   The interior of the can should be clean and free from rust (sulphiding can be ignored apart from trimming).
(10) The odour should be pleasant and correspond to the advertised contents.
(11) The appearance of the contents should be normal.
(12) There should be no disintegration of the contents.
(13) There should be no souring.
(14) There should be no evidence of mould growth.

Elementary principles of bacon curing

The process of producing bacon falls into three distinct operations: (1) slaughtering, (2) carcass preparation and (3) curing.

Slaughtering

Bacon pigs require a few specialised techniques in addition to the standard process of slaughtering and dressing of pork pigs, and it is these additional techniques that will now be described.

Bacon pigs are usually selected between the weight range 63–90 kg (140–200 lb) live weight according to whether the carcass is for the Wiltshire Bacon trade or the heavy hog bacon process.

Immediately after scalding at approximately 60°C (140°F) and dehairing, the carcass is either immersed in a tank of boiling water for 5–10 seconds or passed through a brick-lined burner fired by oil. The object of these processes is to tenderise the rind. This aids the actual cutting of bacon on retail sale and also tends to 'tighten up' the whole carcass, i.e. flanks, hocks, etc. After passing through the burner, the carcasses go through a machine known as a black scraper. The head is partially removed by a cut extending from ear to ear through the neck and pharynx. At this point the head is 'jointed' from the cervical vertebrae at the atlanto-occipital joint. An incision is made down the mid-line of the back of the pig, cutting on to the dorsal spines of the vertebrae. The object is to enter the periosteum on either side of the spines ('fins') where a blunt-spiked instrument is inserted and forced down each side between the bone and the periosteum, thus skinning out the dorsal spines. This process is known as 'finning'.

During splitting the vertebral body is removed by sawing or chopping down each side of the vertebral column leaving only the seven cervical vertebrae intact but split centrally.

The leaf (peritoneal) fat and psoas muscles (undermeat) are removed by cutting and lifting while the carcass is still hot. After a cooling period, usually overnight, the carcass is 'fridged'. The object is to obtain a carcass temperature that does not exceed 3.3–4.4°C (38–40°F). This is of the utmost importance as inadequate cooling before curing is the main cause of tainted shoulders and gammons in the finished product.

The pig carcasses before entering the hanging area are graded. The Wiltshire side is selected broadly into three grades, each of which is further divided for payment purposes. Selection is based upon a combination of carcass length, and leanness, and Fig. 19.1 illustrates the points on a carcass at which measurements are taken. Fixed minimum and maximum measurement standards are laid down for the following points:

(1) Shoulder back fat measurement
(2) Loin back fat measurement
(3) Length of carcass from the symphysis pubis to the 1st rib

A carcass must conform to all three measurement standards to qualify for a particular grade.

The intrascope

In addition to the three external measurements as set out above, by use of an optical instrument known as an intrascope it is now possible to make internal measurements. The probe of the instrument is inserted through the skin and it is then possible visibly to define the division between the 'eye of lean' or longissimus dorsi muscle and back fat, thus giving an accurate back fat measurement. This measurement is written on the leg or shoulder. There are three probing points: 4.5 cm, 67.5 cm and 8 cm from the mid-line of the vertebral dorsal processes in line with the head of the last rib. The 6.5-cm probe measurement is used alone for bacon pigs. The average of the 4.5-cm and 8-cm measurements is used for pork pigs and cutters. A combination of the three readings is useful in detecting any 'shallowing off' or concave effect of the muscle that sometimes occurs in fat pigs.

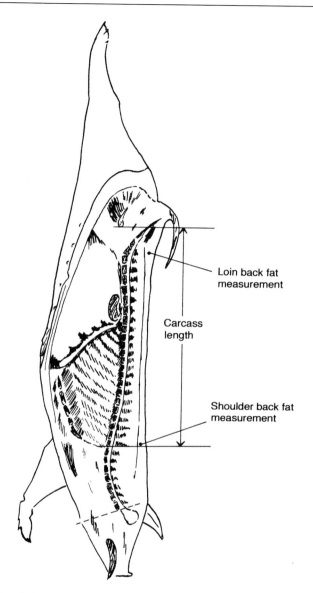

Loin back fat
measurement

Carcass
length

Shoulder back fat
measurement

Fig. 19.1   Grading of pig.

Carcass preparation *(Wiltshire sides)*

The preparation of bacon is usually carried out on a line conveyor system. A series of operations is carried out by each individual.

The side of pork is placed rind down on the conveyor and the feet are removed (Fig. 19.2).

A saw cut is made vertically down through the pelvis to the acetabulum and

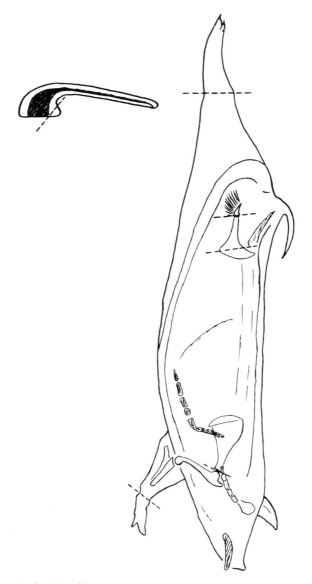

Fig. 19.2 Preparation for side of bacon.

also at a 45° angle through the hip region of the ilium towards the leg. This facilitates the removal of the ilium shaft.

The remains of the vertebral bodies are sawn off at an angle of 45° to the horizontal as in Fig. 19.2, and the tail, 1st rib, sternum and cervical vertebrae are removed.

The scapula must also be pulled out and this is achieved by making an incision down into the scapulo-humeral joint (shoulder joint), severing the scapula from the humerus. A chisel is then introduced into the opened joint and with a gouging action the shoulder muscles are removed from each surface of the scapula. A mechanical extractor attached to the neck of the scapula then removes the intact bone from the shoulder pocket.

The side is now generally trimmed, particular attention being paid to the tail area, back fat, and the neck, which is rounded off removing most of the collar fat. The remains of the diaphragm (skirt) is removed, as also is any loose carcass tissue. Many companies wash the sides to remove the bone dust, and chill a second time to ensure the required temperature before curing. The conversion of pork to bacon yields 80% of the original carcass weight.

Bacon cuts (Fig. 19.3)
Seasonal demand for particular bacon cuts, e.g. summer demand for green gammons, and changing consumer trends for more convenient high quality gammon, back or middle cuts of bacon, has altered the trade. This has tended to lead bacon producers away from the traditional Wiltshire sides to the curing of

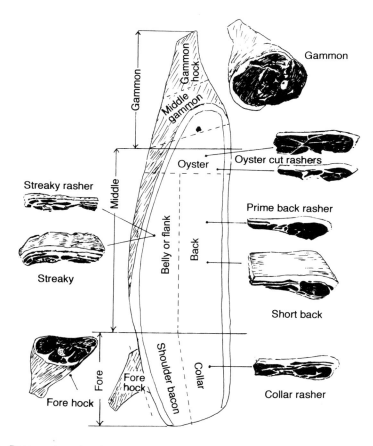

Fig. 19.3   Bacon cuts and rashers.

individual high demand cuts. Some advantages accrue from this, e.g. it reduces the stocks of unsold low demand bacon cut and thus the producer is able to direct these portions into other commodities in the form of fresh pork.

Gammons, middles and fore ends of bacon are obtained from Wiltshire sides. A combination of gammon and middle is known as a threequarter side, and a combination of a fore end and middle as a spencer. A short middle is a middle less the oyster cut. Gammons and short middles are predominant in bacon production.

Prepared pre-cured bacon cuts, as in Wiltshire sides, are washed before curing.

Curing

The curing of bacon as we know it today, i.e. mild tank-cured Wiltshire bacon, was invented by the Danes, but there is evidence that preserving by means of salt alone was practised by the ancients. Dry-curing is still in use today, but has only a limited retail sale.

The principles of bacon curing, whether wet or dry, are:

(1)   To extract moisture from the tissues.
(2)   To replace moisture with salt, which will prevent or retard the growth of putrefactive organisms.

The strength or concentration of salt present in the tissues controls the length of the preserved life. However, nowadays, the pleasing taste of mild bacon is of prime importance. Therefore the mild tank-cured or Danish bacon has a relatively short shelf-life outside refrigeration.

The salt solution replaces the moisture of the tissues by a process of osmosis. The strong salt solution inhibits the growth and multiplication of micro-organisms. There are, however, certain organisms known as salt-tolerant micro-organisms, which feed on exuded proteins and are able to remain active in the brine solution.

Curing can be divided into four stages: (1) pumping, (2) brine immersion, (3) maturing and (4) drying or smoking.

It is important to note that curers employ different methods to produce a commodity suitable for their particular trade, and that therefore curing techniques vary accordingly. There are two types of brine employed in curing: (1) pumping brine and (2) cover or immersion brine. All brines are basically water, salt and nitrite but other additives may include sugar and herbs.

(1)   Pumping brine is generally a saturated salt solution including nitrite and should give a Twaddell Hydrometer reading at 47–48°.
(2)   Cover brine is also a solution of salt, water and nitrite but is weaker than the pumping brine.

In the past, potassium nitrate (saltpetre) was used extensively without control or restriction in brines. Nitrate is reduced to nitrite by salt-tolerant micro-organisms. The nitrite reacts with haemoglobin to form nitroso-haemoglobin, which gives bacon its pink colour. However, it is now known that nitrates and nitrites in high quantities are a health risk. The levels in brine are restricted by legislation.

Hand pumping

The brine is introduced into the prepared side of pork by a series of injections, as indicated in Fig. 19.4. A set pattern is desirable and in each spot a quantity of pumping brine is injected under pressure into the muscle tissue. Care must be taken to see that excessive pressure is not created as this opens up seams and damages carcass tissue.

The process of hand-pumping Wiltshire sides is highly skilled and time con-suming, and for this reason is only found today in small bacon factories. In larger production factories automatic brine pumping machines are used. The uncured sides or individual major cuts move along a conveyor belt and the brine is injected through multiholed injection needles. The needles move vertically up and down. Should a needle come into contact with bone and penetration is checked, the needle remains in the high position.

Owing to the variation in thickness of the sides and the use of multiholed needles, there is an excessive use of brine. Excess brine is collected, filtered and recycled. Brine is introduced into the tissues to a maximum holding capacity and so tank immersion times have been cut dramatically.

Brine immersion (hand pumped Wiltshire sides)

Before being placed in the empty vats the sides have a measure of salt put into the scapula pocket. The sides are stacked in the vats as shown in Fig. 19.4 and sprinkled with a quantity of salt. When the vat is three-quarters full, the cover brine is pumped into the vat and the sides are battened down. Care must be taken not to overfill the vat with sides as this prevents adequate circulation, particularly to the thicker cuts, i.e. the shoulders and gammons, which tend to come into contact with each other.

The sides are kept in the cover brine for 5 days; during this time the process of osmosis takes place.

Multineedle injected sides or cuts are placed in vats for periods as short as 24 hours before being removed and drained for 48 hours.

Maturing

Hand-pumped Wiltshire sides are removed from the vats after 5 days and stacked with the rinds uppermost to drain and mature at a cellar temperature of 5.5°C (42°F) for a further 8–10 days to develop colour and flavour. After 10 days the bacon is in a 'green state' (the trade name for wet, mature bacon), and can be sold as such.

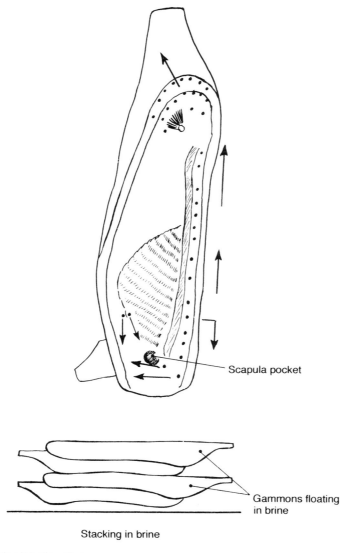

Stacking in brine

Fig. 19.4   Brine injection sites.

Drying or smoking
The bacon may be further dried by hanging in a drying room at 10–15.5°C (50–60°F) for 2–3 days,. This removes the excess moisture and the sides are then sold as pale dried or dry bacon.

The sides can also be smoked after the 'green' stage by being placed in smoke kilns, where oak sawdust smoke is introduced. This adds a distinct flavour and also preserves the sides for a longer period by reducing the liquid content. The smoke also contains acids that are in themselves preservatives in that they exert an antiseptic action.

Bulk transporting

The practice of baling a number of Wiltshire sides in hessian for transporting has been superseded by using disposable heavy-duty cardboard cartons on pallets known as jumbo packs. Each box contains approximately 900 kg (2000 lb) of bacon sides or cuts that should be held at a temperature not exceeding 4°C (39°F).

Dry curing

The dry curing of bacon is based on the same principles as wet curing, i.e. withdrawal of some of the moisture from the tissues and replacement by salt in sufficient concentration to prevent the growth of micro-organisms.

In dry curuing this is achieved by placing a mixture of salt and nitrite on the cut surface of the meat being cured. When curing gammons they are so placed that the cut surfaces are uppermost. This ensures that there is a natural gravitational pull from the cut surfaces down to the hocks. The salt–nitrite mixture diffuses through the muscular tissue by osmosis and thus the desired concentration of salt is achieved.

In the preparation of the gammon, pre-chilling and conditions free from contamination apply, as in the tank-cured bacon.

The time necessary for the process to be complete varies according to the size and type of the cut to be cured. A shoulder belly takes about 14 days and a leg of pork cut to York ham specifications 28–30 days at a cellar temperature of 4.4–5.5°C (40–42°F).

After curing in the cellar the commodity is washed free of salt and nitrite and hung to mature in a dry, airy atmosphere free from flies and other forms of contamination.

The manufacture of sausage

Sausage manufacture is divided into two main types: (1) uncooked, e.g. pork and beef sausages, and (2) cooked, e.g. polonies and liver sausages.

Pork and beef sausages

The manufacture of sausages to the small trader is an operation specifically designed for utilising joints unsold after a week's trading, and it is for this reason that the shelf-life of this particular type of production is relatively short. However, sausage manufacture to the commercial wholesaler is a highly specialised technique designed to produce a commodity for a very competitive market, containing a high percentage of meat, exhibiting a good attractive colour and with a long shelf-life. The attractive colour and long shelf-life depend largely on a low bacterial count and the necessary care during the life of the commodity to minimise the multiplication of the bacteria present.

Heat is a particularly important point for it is heat that allows the multiplication of organisms to accelerate. It is therefore important at all stages during the manufacture of a sausage that the temperature of the commodity be held as low as possible. The post-slaughter temperature of the meat should be 1.1–3.3°C (34–38°F). This should be maintained throughout the boning process. During chopping, which inevitably produces heat by friction, the heat should be checked by the use of flaked ice or chilled water instead of tap water. The chopping should be done speedily so that the temperature of the sausage meat does not rise above 7.2°C (45°F).

Preservatives may also be used in sausages to help the keeping qualities. The practice is strictly controlled by legislation which allows the use of sulphur dioxide at 450 parts per million.

Sausage ingredients

(1) Pork – lean and fat in the ratio of 2:1 and in a pork sausage 65% of the total product.
(2) Rusk.
(3) Water.
(4) Seasonings (including preservative).
(5) Colouring.

Seasonings vary considerably but most contain: white pepper, mace, nutmeg, ginger, cayenne and salt. Powdered milk and blood plasma are often added as binders.

Method of preparation

The defatted pork, back fat, rusk, water and seasoning should be weighed separately and conveniently situated near the bowl chopper. With the machine operating, the defatted meat should be put in first, followed by the seasoning evenly distributed, and then half the cooled water (or flaked ice). The rusk in a dry state is then added, quickly followed by the remaining water and then lastly the fat. The whole operation is carried out at a slow chopping speed within 2.5 minutes and under a sausage meat temperature on extraction of 7.2°C (45°F).

The sausage meat is then filled into casings and linked. This operation produces more heat and introduces some water – the heat from the pressurised filling and the water from the soaked hog or sheep casings. The linked sausage is then passed through a sausage cooler which chills and dries it. At this stage the sausage is usually packed and stored under refrigeration before sale.

Casings

The casings in general use are pig or sheep small intestines that have been cleansed and processed so that only the fibrous or areolar layer remains. The sheep casings or 'skins' are smaller than the pig casings. Casings are graded into small, medium and wide sizes. Sheep casings usually give 16–18 links to 0.5 kg of sausage with an average diameter of 1.5 cm. Pig casings give 6–8 links to 0.5 kg and average up to 2.5 cm in diameter.

Most of the sheep casings used in this country are New Zealand and Australian casings. They are made up in bundles totalling about 90 m in length. Recently there has been a marked increase in the use of synthetic casings since techniques in their development are improving.

Polony

This commodity is an example of a cooked sausage that contains seven parts of pork, three parts back fat, one part rice flour, one part fine white rusk, water and seasoning. The seasoning consists of salt, white pepper, mace, nutmeg, coriander and cinnamon.

Method
The polony meat is chopped in the same way as sausage meat, i.e. the lean meat is added first to the bowl chopper, followed by the seasoning, water, scalded rice flour and lastly the fat. Polony meat is chopped very finely and then filled into extra wide pig casings. It is then tied into large loops about 15 cm in diameter and cooked at a temperature of 76.6°C (170°F) for 25 minutes. After cooking, the polonies are dyed in a standard red polony dye and then transferred from the hot dye liquid into a bath of cold salt water for fixing. They are then placed under refrigeration.

Black pudding

A readily available by-product of the bacon factory or slaughterhouse is blood and this forms the basic ingredient of black puddings.

The blood to be used for black pudding must be defibrinated on collection by stirring to prevent clotting or treated with an anticoagulant, e.g. sodium citrate. This is added to fresh blood in liquid or powder form.

The ingredients of black pudding include 16 parts pig blood, 2 parts pearl barley (pre-cooked for 4 hours), 1.75 parts flour, 1.75 parts fine oatmeal, 1 part onion, seasoning and 8 parts back fat diced into 0.5-cm cubes.

Method
The onions are minced and mixed in a container with the flour, oatmeal, seasoning and pearl barley. The blood is then added with the diced fat and further mixed.

The mixture is filled into cylindrical synthetic casings. After washing in cold water, the puddings are cooked at a temperature of 82.2–87.7°C (180–190°F) for 35 minutes by which time they are quite firm.

The seasoning usually consists of pepper, mixed herbs and nutmeg, plus salt to taste.

Tripe dressing

The ox stomach consists of rumen, reticulum, omasum and abomasum. The rumen and reticulum are most commonly utilised in the form of seam and honeycomb tripe, respectively. The omasum and abomasum are difficult to clean and are brown in colour when processed; they are rarely seen on sale. The oesophagus is sometimes processed and is known as weasand tripe.

Processing

The rumen and reticulum are washed thoroughly as quickly as possible after slaughter and opened out to allow defatting. The black mucous membrane is removed by scalding in hot water, including soda at 60°C (140°F) and scraping by hand or machine. After further washing the stomach is placed in a boiler and cooked until tender. This usually takes up to 4 hours.

The cooked tender stomach is placed in cold water and then the outer peritoneal membrane is removed by brushing. This also serves to remove untrimmed abdominal fat.

The stomach after cooking is not a good colour – usually green or dark grey. This is rectified by bleaching in a solution of cold water and bleaching agent.

Storage of the finished commodity for short periods is best done in chilled water.

As an alternative to scalding to remove the mucous membrane, a lime process can be used.

Chitterlings

Included under the heading of tripe is the relatively uncommon commodity chitterlings.

Chitterlings are processed from the pig's stomach and intestines. Their slow disappearance from the retail trade is due to the care and work that is necessary to clean this commodity entirely from stomach and intestinal contents. The work is therefore exacting and time consuming and most processors prefer to utilise the pig's intestine for sausage casings.

Lard

Leaf (peritoneal) fat and back fat are most commonly used. The technique of rendering lard is simple but the refining requires great care if the end product is to be a first-class pure white lard.

Method

A small quantity of lard from a previous cooking and some water are put into a steam-jacketed pan. To this are added the diced or minced leaf fat and back fat.

Heat is applied and the mixture is stirred regularly. Cooking continues until the fat shows signs of browning. The liquid is then removed into a second cool steam pan.

The refining is done by using a mixture of water and soda, or water, soda and pearl ash. This is added to the reheated lard on the simmer while stirring vigorously. After eliminating the heat and allowing the lard to settle, the dirt and impurities rise to the surface in the form of a scum that is readily skimmed off. The lard is then run into containers and allowed to set.

The residue is pressed to extract all the lard and the remains are either sold as 'scratchings' or used in the manufacture of fertiliser.

Pork brawn

This is a commodity utilising pig head meat in association with lean pork and is therefore a cheap but very palatable product.

The pigs' heads usually without the cheek meat (which is used to produce Bath chaps) are placed in brine at a density of 33° Twaddell hydrometer reading for 4–5 days, after which they are removed and washed thoroughly in cold water.

Method
The heads are then placed in a steam-jacketed pan and cooked for 1.5–2 hours, by which time the bones can be removed easily. The meat is then proportioned, lean in equal proportion to fat. If all the ft head meat is to be used, then lean pork must be added at the brining stage. The meat is then diced or minced according to the desired texture and returned to the boiler containing a quantity of stock from the cooking (usually about 25% of the finished product). After further cooking the seasoning and colouring are added together with previously prepared gelatine if the product has failed to yield sufficient jelly to allow for adequate setting.

The product is then put into moulds and cooled. An occasional stir is necessary to give an even distribution of meat and fat content.

Salt should be added separately to taste owing to the variation of the brine content. The seasoning consists of white pepper, cayenne and mace.

Cooked ham and ox tongue

Certain pork and beef commodities are prepared, cooked and sold in a cold-pressed condition. Such products include ham and ox tongue that are already cured or are cured before cooking.

Cooked ham

The ham in the 'green' state is boned completely and trimmed to remove excess fat. The majority of the rind is left on. The ham is placed rind uppermost in a ham press. The lid of this works on a spring and ratchet system and is forced down on to the ham. There are varying methods of cooking. The commonest is probably the insulated container method. The moulds are placed in the cooker and the water is heated to 82.2°C (180°F). The insulated lid is bolted down and the heat turned off. The cooker retains the desired temperature for 12–14 hours by which time the hams are cooked and tender. The moulds are removed from the cooker, drained and further pressure exerted. When cold and set, the hams are taken from the presses, the rinds removed and a ham dressing applied.

Ox tongues

These are first cured by needle injection and immersion in brine or by arterial pumping into the lingual artery and immersing for up to 6 days. The tongue is cooked by simmering for 3 hours. The tongue 'root' and the hyoid bones are removed and the mucous membrane stripped from the surface. A number of tongues are pressed together, including a gelatine glaze.

Pork pies

Preparation is important in the manufacture of pork pies, e.g. the pastry must be made and adequately rested, the meat boned and processed, seasonings thoroughly mixed and a jelly prepared, which is held at 65.5–82°C (150–180°F) until used.

Pie cases were originally 'pulled up' by hand round a wooden mould. However, today the commonest method is cold pastry moulding in tins on specially designed machines that press out the pie case, deposit the required weight of meat into the case and press fix the lid.

The pie, still in a metal container, is cooked in an oven at a temperature of 204.5°C (400°F) for 35–60 minutes according to size.

Jellying is done immediately after cooking by needle injection when the hot meat absorbs a quantity of the liquor and swells accordingly. A second jellying should be done when cold to fill complet ely and seal the pie.

Pastry preparation
Ingredients – flour, lard, salt and water. The lard and salt are mixed well in a bowl mixer and the flour thoroughly 'rubbed in'. The water, either hot or cold, is added last. The pastry is allowed to 'rest' for about an hour before use.

Meat preparation
Pork should be selected – leg, shoulder and belly draft in the ratio 1:2, fat to lean. The meat is then minced or chopped to the desired texture and transferred to a bowl mixer where the seasoning, binder (in the form of rusk or rice cones) and

water are added. The meat is placed quickly under refrigeration if not intended to be used immediately.

Pie meat seasoning preparation

The seasoning is thoroughly mixed and salt added. The mixture contains 3 kg salt, 1 kg white pepper, 90 g cayenne, 60 g nutmeg and 60 g mace; 150 g of the above mixture is added to 4.5 kg of prepared meat.

Jelly preparation

Most manufacturers use a branded manufactured gelatine – usually 60 g to 1 litre of boiling water, plus a seasoning to taste. However, a cheap and efficient jelly can be produced from feet and rinds. The preparation involves a thorough washing, brining overnight, followed by a thorough washing in the morning. The product is then simmered at 99.9°C (210°F) for 5–6 hours. It is important not to boil as calcium separates out and clouds the end product. The liquor is then removed and simmered in a second boiler until a thicker gelatinous consistency is produced. The seasoning is added and setting quality checked.

Chapter 20
Food Poisoning from Meat Products

Spoilage and putrefaction of meat are not in themselves harmful. It is equally clear, however, that illness may result from eating meat containing any number of harmful agents. Such agents may be inorganic chemical substances, certain animal parasites and micro-organisms, including bacteria, or their toxic products. Of the agents, bacteria and their toxins are undoubtedly responsible for the greatest number of food-poisoning cases. The resulting diseases, which comprise several different types of illness, may be conveniently divided into two classes:

(1) Infections in which living bacteria are necessary for the development of the disease.
(2) Intoxications, in which products of the bacteria are responsible.

Food poisoning caused by living agents

Campylobacter

Until the late 1970s *Campylobacter* species were only associated with diarrhoea and abortion in cattle and sheep. It was then recognised to be a cause of food poisoning in humans and it is now the most common reported cause of food-borne infection, surpassing even the *Salmonella* species. It is a commensal of cattle, sheep, birds, fowl, rodents and domestic pets such as cats and dogs. Many of these animals are asymptomatic carriers and are the reservoirs for human infection resulting from the consumption of contaminated food, i.e. poultry, milk and water. Unpasteurised milk or milk used from bottles the tops of which have been pecked by birds is the most common reported food vehicle.

Campylobacter jejuni is the most common species identified in human infection. Clinically it has the same features of many food poisoning bacteria and so it cannot be diagnosed on clinical grounds alone. The illness occurs between 2–10 days after exposure and may last for a week or more. The symptoms include a profuse diarrhoea which may contain fresh blood, nausea but rarely vomiting, severe abdominal cramps and fever.

Infections of *Campylobacter* have been associated with subsequent illness in cases of Guillain–Barré syndrome.

Listeria monocytogenes (see p. 129)

Salmonella (see salmonellosis, pp. 132, 274)
These are a group of bacteria of more than 2200 types or species, commonly known as the paratyphoid bacteria. They inhabit the intestine of animals, including humans.

Some of the salmonella group produce a typhoid-like febrile disease in humans that can be diagnosed only by isolating the specific organism. Others commonly produce the more usual gastroenteritis. They have to be living to cause either of these diseases, since bacteria-free filtrates of cultures or heat-killed organisms do not produce illness.

Typical food poisoning commences within 7–72 hours after ingesting the organisms and is characterised by nausea, vomiting, abdominal pains and diarrhoea. The severity of the disease differs in different outbreaks and among various individuals in the same outbreak. Old people and young babies are particularly vulnerable to food poisoning. The meat involved is often derived from infected animals, especially calves, pigs and poultry, but the meat may be contaminated during storage or preparation by infected humans or animals, including rats and mice. Contaminated foods have no abnormal odour or taste.

It is important to remember that healthy animals may be carriers of salmonellae. The bacteria in these cases are present only in small numbers, and if the meat is properly refrigerated and cooked no ill effects follow.

Many cases of salmonella food poisoning occur at Christmas time due to the increased consumption of poultry, especially frozen turkeys. Frozen poultry must be thoroughly thawed prior to cooking and the meat must be thoroughly cooked. To check that the meat is thoroughly cooked the thickest parts of the flesh on the breast and legs of the poultry should be checked with a skewer to see if the meat juices run clear.

Salmonellae grow well on meat at ordinary room temperature. They are not destroyed by freezing or in the usual pickling solutions, but are killed by the temperatures attained in commercial pasteurisation and in the processing of canned goods.

The most common cause of food poisoning from salmonella is *Salmonella enteritidis*, with the *PT4* phagetype the most common of these. *Salmonella enteritidis* PT4 is associated with poultry and eggs. *Salmonella enteritidis* is a notifiable disease and any egg-producing flocks found to be affected are slaughtered. It has also been isolated from cattle, pigs, goats and ducks. The second most common salmonella is *S. typhimurium*, which has also been isolated from cattle, sheep, pigs, fowl and ducks.

Yersinia enterocolitica
This bacterium is found widely amongst wild and domestic animals. It causes infection in humans by the consumption of contaminated food or water. The symptoms include diarrhoea, abdominal pain, fever, headache, pharyngitis,

acute mesenteric lymphadenitis, pseudo appendicitis, vomiting and arthritis. It has an incubation period of between 1–5 days. *Yersinia* is able to grow readily on meat under refrigeration and competes with the normal bacterial flora on the meat.

Food poisoning caused by bacillary toxins

Certain bacteria may produce toxins when growing on food. These toxins are extremely irritant to the human intestine. Symptoms are apparent 2–3 hours after ingestion (cf. the 7–72 hours of salmonella food poisoning) and persist for 8–24 hours. It is rarely, if ever, fatal and generally of very brief duration.

Bacteria in this type of food poisoning are *Staphylococcus aureus*, *Proteus*, streptococci, *E. coli* and *Clostridium perfringens*. The toxins of these bacteria are present in meat before it is eaten. They are very resistant to heat and some have withstood boiling for 30 minutes.

The toxin-producing bacteria may be present in the animal before it is slaughtered and the meat is thus contaminated at the source, but meat is often contaminated from extraneous sources, e.g. from humans with septic sore throats, septic wounds (especially of the hands), etc.

Botulism
This is a very dangerous form of food poisoning with a high mortality. It is caused by the toxins produced by various strains of *Clostridium botulinum* (from the Latin *botulinus* – a sausage), an anaerobic spore-forming bacillus. There are five main strains, with types A, B and E causing botulism in humans, and types C and D in animals. The toxins are neurotrophic (affinity for nerves) and symptoms commence within 12–36 hours. These are lassitude, headaches and giddiness leading to paralysis. Very often there is only very slight or even no intestinal disturbance. The toxins are destroyed by cooking, and botulism in humans is generally associated with pickled or smoked foods that have been allowed to stand for a period and then not cooked properly. In the Loch Maree outbreak in Scotland in 1922, all eight people who ate potted wild duck paste sandwiches died within 7 days. In Birmingham in 1978 four people contracted the disease after eating tinned salmon contaminated with *Clostridium botulinum* type E. In spite of intensive care, two of the four died.

Botulism is well known as a disease of ducks and other water-fowl. In 1969 two outbreaks occurred in Coventry and Leicester causing hundreds of deaths in various types of ducks and in swans, coots and moorhens.

Botulism occurs in many species of animals and birds. Cases have occurred in cattle, with a high mortality rate. In one case the cattle had been fed on ensiled poultry litter. Post-mortem findings were enlarged spleen, congestion of the intestinal mucosae, and petechiae in various organs and tissues.

In zoos, lions have been affected by being fed on carcasses of casulty broiler chickens, monkeys from contaminated fowl carcasses, and birds from being fed on commercially bred maggots.

Judgement: Reject whole carcass, offal and blood.

Escherichia coli (E. coli)

Most strains of this bacterium are harmless, being commensals in both animal and human intestines. Some strains cause illness by different infective and toxin-producing mechanisms. The most famous of these is *E. coli* O157 which was identified in the early 1980s but is still a relatively uncommon cause of food poisoning with reported cases reaching an estimated 1000 in the UK for 1996.

The reason for this particular strain's notoriety is its relatively high fatality rate of 1–5%, the severity of the illness and the long-term medical consequences, especially in children. These can include kidney failure.

E. coli O157 has had strong media coverage following the Lanarkshire outbreak in November 1996 and the Japanese outbreak in May 1996. However, it has been the cause of many major outbreaks in the USA since the 1980s. In the Lanarkshire outbreak, 18 elderly people died of the 285 confirmed cases.

The most common source of *E. coli* O157 is healthy cattle, but research in 1996 has shown sheep to be a source also. Other strains of *E. coli* are also pathogenic to humans. The symptoms for all strains are watery or prolonged diarrhoea, nausea, abdominal cramps, fever and, rarely, vomiting. The incubation period is between 12 and 72 hours with a duration of up to 7 days.

Most cases are associated with the consumption of undercooked minced beef products such as beefburgers and raw milk. However, other outbreaks have been linked to raw vegetables, unpasteurised apple juice and water. The method of transmission is contamination by gut contents at slaughter, by manure or by contact with the animals.

The Advisory Committee on the Microbiological Safety of Food in 1995 indicated that one of the control measures to prevent such illness was the need to minimise the contamination of carcasses at slaughter. Even minor contamination is a problem as the effective dose of *E. coli* O157 is very low, probably less than 100 organisms.

In the USA a carcass steam pasteurisation system which is designed to be installed immediately after the carcass wash in the slaughterhouse has been undergoing full-scale trials following successful laboratory tests. The system is split into three stages. The first stage is designed to remove surface water from the carcass. The second stage is a steam chamber where steam pasteurises the surface by raising the surface temperature to 85°C for 8 seconds. The final stage is when the carcass is rapidly chilled with water sprays.

Rabbits

Chapter 21
Diseases of Rabbits

The wild rabbit population of Britain was virtually wiped out by myxomatosis, which appeared in 1953, but has now recovered to record levels. Since 1953 the majority of rabbit meat eaten in this country has been imported frozen from China, Australia and Poland. However, an increasing number of rabbits are now being intensively produced here. The commonest breeds are the New Zealand White and the Californian. Crosses of the two breeds are common and give an optimum live weight of 2–2.5 kg at 14 weeks. There is a 35% loss of weight during dressing of the carcass.

Rabbits are usually stunned by electricity and then killed by dislocation of their necks. They are skinned, the head is removed and their are eviscerated. The carcasses are cooled by cold water or ice sludge.

The disease pattern has altered as it has done with other intensively produced animals and poultry.

Atrophic rhinitis

See pasteurellosis (p. 232).

Coccidiosis

There are two types, hepatic coccidiosis and intestinal coccidiosis.

(1) The hepatic type is caused by *Eimeria stiedae*. The liver becomes very much enlarged with distended bile ducts, which appear as yellowish white lesions filled with a pus-like material [Plate 4(b)]. Petechial haemorrhages may be widespread throughout the viscera and carcass, which may be emaciated and oedematous. The liver is rejected.
    Judgement: Dependent upon the state of the carcass.
(2) The intestinal type is caused by *Eimeria irresidua*, *E. magna* and *E. perforans*. The duodenum becomes enlarged and contains a whitish mucus. There are petechial haemorrhages in the caecum.
    Judgement: The carcass is passed unless there is emaciation.

Coenurus serialis

See tapeworms (p. 146).

Contagious catarrh

See 'snuffles' (p. 233).

Cysticerus pisiformis

See tapeworms (p. 146).

Gastroenteritis

This is probably the commonest disease of rabbits and inclues mucoid enteritis. Many factors and bacteria have been implicated. Post-mortem lesions are variable but frequently there is a diffuse enteritis with watery intestinal contents.

Judgement: Depends upon the state of the carcass.

Myxomatosis

This is caused by a virus spread by the rabbit flea, *Spylopsyllus cuniculi*. The symptoms of the disease are characteristic. There is a discharge from the eyes that is clear at first but later becomes thicker. As a result thick crusts and swellings appear around the eyes. Fleshy tumours develop in various parts of the body and cause large swellings at the base of the ears, on the nose, under the chin and around the anus and genitals. The disease is not transmissible to humans.

Judgement: Total rejection.

Nephritis

This is a common condition in rabbits caused by *Toxoplasma gondii*. The carcass is generally congested and sets badly. The carcass lymph nodes are enlarged and oedematous. The most striking lesions are in the kidneys, which are enlarged and contain circumscribed irregular greyish areas and in chronic cases pitted areas.

Judgement: Carcasses are very often emaciated and should be rejected.

Parasitic gastroenteritis

This is caused by a roundworm, *Graphidium strigosum*. The male is 8–6 mm and the female 11–20 mm long. Heavy infestations may cause diarrhoea and emaciation.

Another roundworm, *Passalurus ambiguus*, occurs in the large intestine but it appears to be relatively harmless.

Judgement: Dependent upon the state of the carcass.

Pasteurellosis or atrophic rhinitis

This disease is caused by *Pasteurella multocida*. It affects the respiratory tract, mainly causing pneumonia. Sometimes the turbinate bones are affected causing atrophic rhinitis.

Judgement: Total rejection.

Rabbit syphilis

This is caused by a spirochaete, *Treponema cuniculi.* The disease takes the form of small papules and moist ulcers on the vulva of the doe and the prepuce of the buck. Spread, however, may take place to the head and hocks and eventually become generalised on the skin of the body. It is not transmissible to humans.

Judgement: Local trimming.

Ringworm

This is fairly common and the lesions are similar to those in other animals (p. 166).

'Snuffles' or contagious catarrh

This is a common respiratory disease of rabbits. The cause is unknown but many different bacteria have been isolated from infected rabbits. These include streptococci, staphylococci, *Pasteurella multocida* and *Bordetella bronchiseptica.* Pneumonia is the common feature and is very similar to the lesions in enzootic pneumonia in pigs. The affected parts of the lungs are sharply demarcated. They are confined to the anterior lobes of the lungs and are firm deep red; a yellowish pus may be expressed from the cut bronchioles. Pleurisy, pericarditis and acute tracheitis may also be present.

Judgement: Dependent upon the state of the carcass.

Sore hocks

These are due to rubbing on the wire floors of cages, etc. Secondary infection can cause a pyaemia with abscesses in the kidneys.

Judgement: Total rejection or local trimming if only the hocks are affected.

Tapeworm cysts

Two types are found in rabbits, *Coenurus serialis* and *Cysticercus pisiformis* (see p. 151).

Tuberculosis

This is very rare in rabbits but they are susceptible to both the bovine and avian strains.

Judgement: Total rejection.

Imported frozen rabbits

In imported frozen rabbits various conditions are encountered.

(1)   Contamination owing to faulty dressing.
(2)   Decomposition.
(3)   Freezer burn (see p. 206).
(4)   Jaundice (see Rimmington and Fowrie test, p. 105).
(5)   Maggots (dead) of *Calliphora vomitoria* and *C. erythrocephala*.
(6)   Mould. This appears as white spots and may be wiped off, but severely affected carcasses should be rejected as they have a musty odour.
(7)   Yellow fat. This is a chemical change that takes place after prolonged refrigeration. It is confined to the surface of the fat. The fat has a rancid smell.

   Judgement: Total rejection in all cases.

Poultry

Chapter 22

Sex and Age Characteristics of Poultry

Poultry are domesticated birds that are bred specifically to provide meat and eggs for human consumption. They include fowl, ducks, geese, turkeys and guinea fowl.

Fowl are the main source of meat and eggs for consumption. They all come from two generic flocks.

(1)   *Chicken or broiler.* Bred for poultry meat production. These birds are specifically bred from the Light Sussex cross for rapid weight gain, white flesh, long body and good breast-meat development. They can be recognised by their white feathers, some of which will remain on the dressed bird. They get the name broiler from the broiler houses in which they are bred. A broiler house can hold up to 20 000 or more birds. They are only 6–8 weeks old at the time of slaughter.

(2)   Hen. Although sold for meat as hens or boiling fowl, they are specifically bred for their egg production capabilities. They are from a Rhode Island Red cross and can be recognised by their red-brown feathers. They are at least 18 months old and display all the secondary sexual and ageing characteristics (see below).

Identification and ageing of poultry

(1) Fowl

It is important to know the differences between the young chickens bred for their meat and the older birds which are bred for their egg production with their meat value being of secondary importance for the producer. The following are the main identification features:

(a) Head
The fowl head has two distinct features which all fowl display. First, they have the comb. This is a fleshy serrated crest beginning at the base of the top beak and running backwards over the crown of the head. Secondly, they have wattles,

which are loose, fleshy, pouch-like bags. One wattle is situated underneath each side of the lower beak.

The hens, being much older, have developed their secondary sexual characteristics.

Old: Comb well developed and is a bright red colour. Wattles well developed. Beak hard and rigid.

Young: Comb poorly developed and is a much lighter colour. Wattles small and under developed. Beak soft and pliable.

(b) Skin
Old: Rough and feather follicles easily visible, especially on the legs. Hair-like feathers (filoplumes) visible, especially on the back of the bird.

Young: Smooth, relatively flawless. Only down feathers visible.

(c) Body
Old: Breast bone protrudes sharply giving a characteristic hatchet-shaped breast. Distended abdomen with large amounts of deposited fat. Breast bone has fully ossified and is hard. Vent is extended and large to allow egg laying.

Young: Broad, well-fleshed breast. No distension of the abdomen. End of breast bone still cartilage (xyphoid) and is soft and pliable. Vent is small.

(d) Legs and feet
Old: Leg scales hard and coarse. Larger feet. Claws large and rigid.

Young: Leg scales soft and smooth. Small feet. Claws shorter and softer.

In addition the intended use for the bird will be determined by the colour of any feathers. White feathers denote a bird intended for meat production; red/brown feathers denote an egg-laying bird.

(2) Turkey

In turkeys it is important to be able to identify the differences between the male and female rather than the age, as in fowl.

The turkey, like the fowl, has two distinct features on its head and neck. First, at the base of the upper beak is a fleshy, finger-like projection called a snood. Secondly, turkeys have numerous wattles on the neck which resemble small fleshy pouches. The head and neck of a turkey have no feathering to cover the skin.

(a) Overall appearance
Male: Longer neck, legs and overall size.

Female: Shorter and more compact.

(b) Sexual characteristics
Male: Has a 'brush', which is a small patch of coarse black hairs at the base of the neck. Snood is longer and thicker. Wattles more developed and the neck skin has a more wrinkled appearance. Older males have spurs on the legs. No feathers seen beyond the neck wattles, only skin.

Female: No 'brush' evident. Snood smaller. Less well developed wattles and smoother neck skin. Only spur buds visible. Line of feathers go up the back of the neck to the base of the skull.

A number of terms are given to poultry, depending on the age and sex of the bird at the time of slaughter. The following terminology is applied to fowl.

Chicken or broiler
This is a young male or female domestic fowl. It has not developed any secondary sexual characteristics as it is usually slaughtered between 6 and 8 weeks of age. It weighs about 2 Kg (4 lbs) and is suitable for roasting.

Petit poussin or poussin
This is an even younger chicken which is slaughtered when weighing about 0.3 kg (0.5 lb). It is also suitable for roasting.

Roaster
This is an older chicken, being up to 8 months of age and weighing about 2.7 kg (6 lb).

Broiler breeder or cob
This is a sexually mature female which has laid fertilised eggs to produce more chickens or broilers. They will be about 18 months of age and weigh about 2.7 kg (6 lb). Normally roasted.

Hen or boiling fowl
This is an egg-laying female bird which has completed at least one egg-laying season. It will be about 18 months of age and has developed all the secondary sexual characteristics. It is not tender enough meat to roast and is boiled to cook it.

Capon
This was a male chicken of 15–16 weeks of age which had been neutered by hormonal implant or surgery. It is now illegal to produce such a bird. However, a similar type of bird is produced without being neutered; it is called a capon-style or *heavy roaster*.

Cockerel

This is a sexually mature male domestic fowl. They are not used for human consumption.

Pullet

This is a young hen.

There are fewer categories of turkey as they are older when slaughtered. This is to give them the time necessary to grow to the larger size and weight demanded by the consumer. The following terminology is applied to turkeys.

Stag

This is a male turkey.

Hen

This is a female turkey.

Poult

This is a young turkey. The term can also be used for young domestic fowl.

Chapter 23
Anatomy of the Fowl

Skin

The skin is composed of two layers, the *epidermis* and the *dermis*. It is usually creamy white and thin. Unlike mammalian skin it has few sebaceous and no sweat glands, but it does have a *uropygeal* or oil gland not present in mammals. This in poultry is small, about 5 mm in diameter, but is much larger in water birds. It lies on the dorsal surface of the tail and has two lobes producing a yellow ceruminous material, which is used in preening the feathers. Other accessory structures of the skin are the slaws, beaks, wattles, combs and ear lobes. The fold of skin filling in the angle between the humerus and radius, i.e. between the body and the wing, is called the *patagium*.

In most areas the skin is covered with feathers, which arise from feather follicles that project into the dermis. Feathers are composed entirely of a horny substance called *keratin*. They fall into three main categories:

(1) Contour feathers.
(2) Downy feathers.
(3) Filoplumes, which are hair-like.

Contour feathers are arranged in rows within areas called *pterylae*. These areas are separated by non-feathered areas called *apteria*. The largest contour feathers are the flight feathers of the wings and the feathers of the tail.

A typical contour feather (Fig. 23.1) consists of a central *shaft* or *rachis*; a lower part, the *calamus* or *quill*; and an upper part or *vane*. At the end of the quill is a small opening, the *inferior umbilicus*. During growth it connects with a papilla of the dermis. The quill is rounded and almost transparent, and contains a series of scales. At the junction of the quill and axis is another small opening, the *superior umbilicus*, from which arises a small additional feather, the *afterfeather*. The axis of the vane, the rachis, has a central groove, and is solid, tapering and flexible.

The vane consists of filaments or *barbs* arising from each side of the rachis at 45° and in turn smaller filaments or *barbules* project distally and proximally also at about 45° (Fig. 23.2). The result is that the barbules cross each other at an angle of about 90°. Hooklets from each set of barbules engage with recesses in corresponding barbules (Fig. 23.2). This interlocking gives firmness to the vane. The

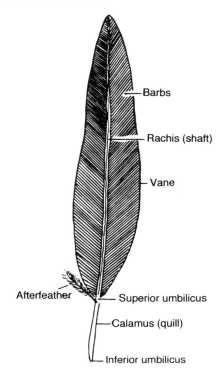

Barbs

Rachis (shaft)

Vane

Afterfeather

Superior umbilicus

Calamus (quill)

Inferior umbilicus

Fig. 23.1 Contour feather.

contour feathers can be raised or depressed by muscles attached to the feather follicles.

Feathers are extremely light in spite of their complex structure and size.

Skeletal system

The *skeleton* (Fig. 23.4) of the fowl differs in certain aspects from that of mammals. The bones are light and some have pneumatic cavities, which may be in direct communication with the respiratory system by way of the air sacs, e.g. humerus and coracoid.

The *skull* bones are fused early in development and hence the sutures are not apparent. The orbits are large. The two premaxillae that form the bony basis of the upper beak are fused as are the dentary parts of the mandibles that form the bony basis of the lower beak. There is only one occipital condyle, which allows for extensive rotation of the head. The whole bony skull is extremely light.

The *vertebral column* consists of the cervical, thoracic, lumbar, sacral, caudal and coccygeal vertebrae. (**NB** Authorities differ in the differentiation of the cervical and thoracic vertebrae.)

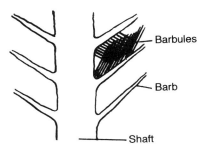

Fig. 23.2 Magnified diagram of feather.

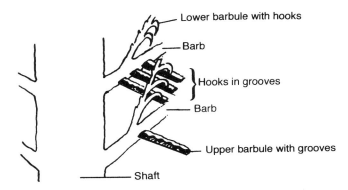

Fig. 23.3 Magnified diagram of interlocking barbules.

(1) The cervical vertebrae number 13 or 14 in the fowl compared with seven in mammals. They form the basis of the very long flexible neck. Except for the atlas, which is very small and ring-like, they have long bodies. The last cervical is often fused with the 1st thoracic vertebra. The last two cervical articulate with the first two ribs.

(2) There are four thoracic vertebrae. The first three are fused together with the last cervical. The 4th thoracic is movable.

(3) The four lumbar, five sacral and six caudal vertebrae are all fused solidly together to form the *synsacrum*. They are also fused with the pelvic bones forming the bony pelvis.

(4) There are six coccygeal vertebrae and these are small except the last – the *pygostyle*, which is flattened laterally.

The vertebral column of the fowl is therefore unlike that of mammals in that the neck portion is extremely flexible while the rest of it is rigid, except at the 4th thoracic vertebra, because of the extensive fusion.

There are seven pairs of *ribs* that articulate with the last two cervical, the four thoracic and the 1st lumbar vertebrae. The first two pairs do not reach the sternum. The other ribs consist of two segments, the vertebral and sternal

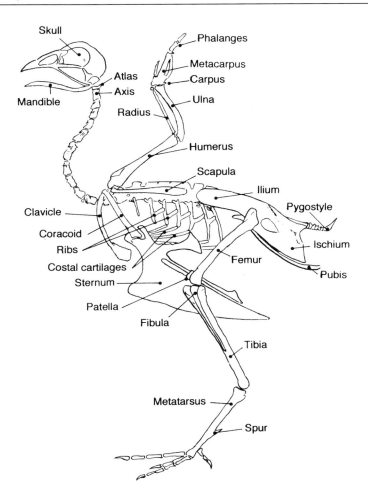

Fig. 23.4 Skeleton of fowl.

segments. The sternal segments articulate with the sternum. With the exception of the 1st and 7th pairs, they all have small flat *uncinate processes* that project backwards over the outer surfaces of the next ribs.

The *sternum* (Fig. 23.5) articulates in front with the coracoids and with the five sternal ribs.

The *pectoral girdle* on each side is composed of the scapula, the coracoid and the clavicle. The fused clavicles are commonly called the 'wishbone'. The bones fit together like a tripod, the coracoids articulating with the sternum at the rostrum. The top of the tripod is the fused ends of the clavicles, which articulate with the humeri.

The *wing* is composed of the humerus, radius and ulna, carpus, metacarpus and the digits.

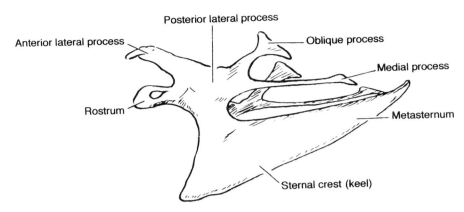

Fig. 23.5 Sternum of fowl.

The *leg* consists of:

(1)   the femur, which articulates with the pelvis at the acetabulum
(2)   the patella, which is small
(3)   the tibia or 'drumstick'
(4)   the fibula, which is slender and pointed with a flattened head and extends three-quarters the length of the tibia
(5)   the metatarsus, on the medial aspect of which, in the male, is a bony projection that bears the spur
(6)   the digits, of which there are four; the 1st digit, which is the only one that projects backwards, has two or three phalanges, the 2nd digit three phalanges, the 3rd four phalanges and the 4th five phalanges. The last phalange on each digit is the core of the nail or claw.

The *pelvic* bones (Fig. 23.6) on each side are the ilium, ischium and pubis. They are fused together and with the synsacrum, i.e. the last thoracic vertebra, the lumbar, sacral and caudal vertebrae form a fused solid complex structure.

The muscular system

This varies in certain aspects from the muscular system of mammals.
The diaphragm is rudimentary and therefore does not divide the body cavity into thoracic and abdominal cavities. It also plays no part in respiration.
The pectoral or breast muscles are very much enlarged. They are lighter in colour (white muscle) than the muscles of the legs. The pectoral muscles are made up of two types of muscle fibres, large and small. The large type, which predominates in the pectoral muscles, is light in colour. The small type is dark. The pectoral muscles make up half the weight of the total musculature. Their function is to depress the wings in flying. The supracoracoid muscles, which raise the wings, are much smaller and are covered by the pectorals.

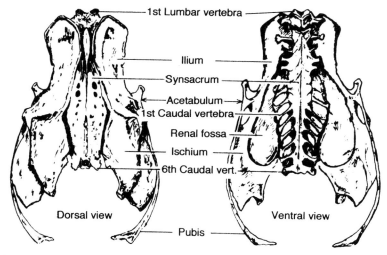

1st Lumbar vertebra

Ilium

Synsacrum

Acetabulum

1st Caudal vertebra

Renal fossa

Ischium

6th Caudal vert.

Dorsal view   Ventral view

Pubis

Fig. 23.6 Pelvic bones of fowl.

The ambiens muscle, which does not occur in mammals, is used in perching. It lies on the medial aspect of the thigh, originates close to the acetabulum and joins the flexor muscles of the digits.

The digestive system

The digestive system (Fig. 23.7) consists of the mouth, tongue, oesophagus, crop, proventriculus, gizzard, duodenum, ileum, caeca, rectum, cloaca and vent. For descriptive purposes liver and spleen are included.

The *mouth* (Fig. 23.8) has no teeth and therefore there is no mastication of food. The grinding up of food takes place in the gizzard. There are no lips or cheeks as in mammals. These are replaced by the beak, which is composed of dense and horny skin covering the mandibles and premaxillae. It is used for picking up and sometimes tearing food. The mouth and tongue have numerous horny papillae directed backwards. The mucous membrane contains numerous glands, which produce mucus. There are no salivary glands. The palate has a long narrow median slit opening into the nasal passages.

The *oesophagus* extends from the pharyngeal area at the back of the mouth to the proventriculus. About one-third of the way down the oesophagus and just before entering the body cavity is the *crop*, used for the temporary storage of food (Fig. 23.9). The oesophageal mucous membrane has numerous glandular cells. These are absent in the crop. The remaining two-thirds of the oesophagus is the thoracic portion and this is in the body cavity. It enters the proventriculus.

The *proventriculus* is the first part of the stomach. It is tubular in shape and smaller than the gizzard. Its mucous membrane has numerous glands producing gastric juice. Before joining the gizzard the proventriculus narrows.

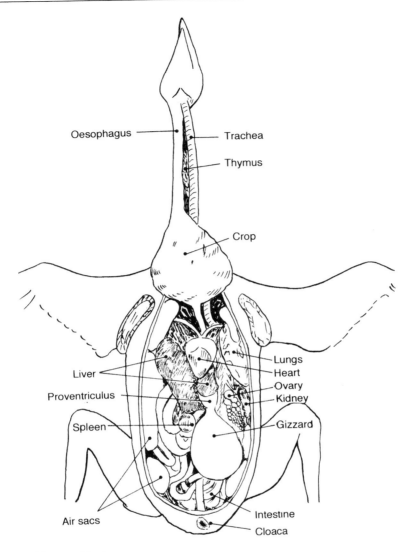

Fig. 23.7 Viscera of fowl.

The *gizzard* is the second part of the stomach. It is very muscular and often contains grit or small stones, which assist in the grinding up of the food. The interior has a pale, ridged, thick and horny lining. Issuing from the gizzard is the first part of the small intestine, the duodenum.

The *duodenum* is a U-shaped loop, between the legs of which is situated the pale-coloured pancreas. The second part of the small intestine is the ileum.

The *ileum* consists of coils or loops suspended from the dorsal wall of the body cavity by the embranous mesentery. The ileum joins the large intestine, which is very similar in diameter to the small intestine. Half way along the ileum is a small diverticulum – the *vitelline diverticulum* – which may become impac-

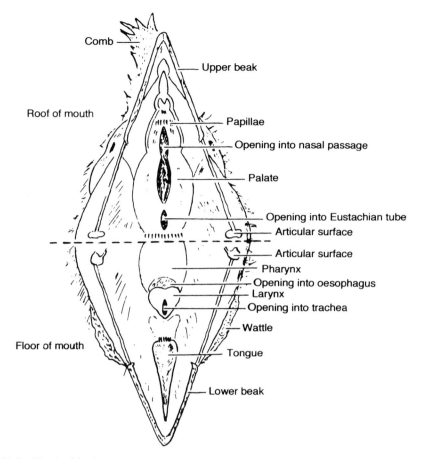

Comb

Upper beak

Roof of mouth

Papillae

Opening into nasal passage

Palate

Opening into Eustachian tube

Articular surface

Articular surface

Pharynx

Opening into oesophagus

Larynx

Opening into trachea

Wattle

Floor of mouth

Tongue

Lower beak

Fig. 23.8   Mouth of fowl.

ted and greatly enlarged. Where the ileum joins the large intestine the caeca
branch off.

The *caeca* or *caecal tubes* (Fig. 23.10) are two blind-ended sacs that project
backwards. They are easily distinguished as their contents are dark in colour. At
the beginning of the caeca, are two small swellings in the mucosa, the so-called
'caecal tonsils'.

The *rectum*, the next part of the large intestine, is short and terminates at the
cloaca.

The *cloaca* (Fig. 23.11) has three parts:

(1)   The *coprodeum* (faecal chamber), which receives the intestinal waste from
the rectum.
(2)   The *urodeum* (urogenital chamber) receives the urates from the kidneys via
the ureters, the eggs in the female via the oviduct and the sperm in the male
via the deferent ducts.

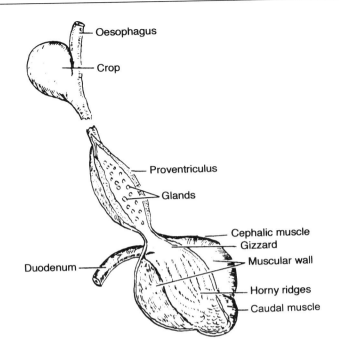

Fig. 23.9 Crop and stomach of fowl.

(3)   The *proctodeum*, which connects with the bursa of Fabricius (cloacal bursa).

The *vent* is the terminal opening of the digestive tract.

The bursa of Fabricius or the cloacal bursa lies dorsal to the cloaca. It is a small spherical glandular sac, which is at its largest in fowls of 3-4 months old. It is part of the lymphatic system and its function is the production of antibodies. It opens into the proctodeum of the cloaca.

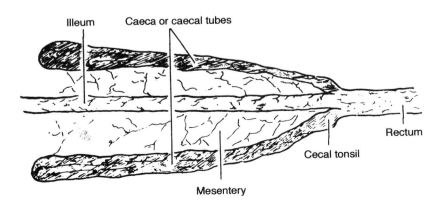

Fig. 23.10   Caeca of fowl.

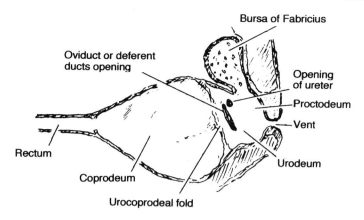

Fig. 23.11 Cloaca.

The *liver* in the fowl is normally of a light chocolate brown colour. This, however, varies greatly, e.g. in very fat hens the liver is very fatty and is yellow. It has two lobes, which are connected by a narrow isthmus. The right lobe is slightly larger than the left. The gall bladder lies on the visceral surface of the right lobe. The left lobe has an independent bile duct conveying bile direct to the intestine and not via the gall bladder.

The *spleen* lies close to the junction of the proventriculus and gizzard. It is small and spherical and because of its bright reddish-brown colour is easily distinguished.

The respiratory system

The external respiratory system in birds consists of the nostrils, nasal cavities, pharynx, larynx, trachea, lungs and air sacs.

The *nostrils*, one on each side of the base of the beak, are rounded or oval openings. They are small and lead into the nasal cavities.

The *nasal cavities* connect with the mouth through an opening in the palate.

The *pharynx* is at the back of the mouth and is not clearly defined.

The *larynx* is heart-shaped. It has no epiglottis or thyroid cartilage and no vocal cords.

The *trachea* has over 100 complete cartilaginous rings. Just before the terminal end of the trachea and just before it bifurcates into two bronchi is the *syrinx* or *lower larynx* or *voice organ*. It appears as a lateral compession of the trachea, inside which are two thin membranes. These are comparable to the vocal cords of mammals. The trachea bifurcates into the right and left bronchi, one going to each lung.

The *lungs* are bright red and positioned in deep recesses formed by the 1st to 5th ribs and are therefore difficult to remove from the body cavity. The dorsal surfaces are deeply grooved by the 2nd, 3rd, 4th and 5th ribs. The ventral surfaces are smooth. Each lung has a primary bronchus, which passes through the lung and leads directly into the large abdominal air sac. From the primary bronchus, secondary and tertiary bronchi spread throughout the lung. The bronchi communicate with the thin-walled air sacs and some of the pneumatic bones.

The *air sacs* are thin walled, transparent and glistening. With the exception of the *clavicular air sac* they are bilateral and paired.

(1)   The *cervical air sacs* lie dorsal to the oesophagus and extend from the 2nd cervical to the 2nd thoracic vertebrae.
(2)   The *clavicular air sac* lies in the anterior part of the body cavity and has diverticula that enter the pneumatic foramena of the humeri.
(3)   The *anterior* and *posterior thoracic air sacs* lie caudally and ventrally to the lungs.
(4)   The *abdominal air sacs* are the largest and cover the viscera from the duodenum backwards.

All the air sacs pass the air back to the trachea so that air only flows one way through the lungs and air sacs.

The circulatory system

The circulatory system in birds follows roughly the same pattern as in mammals. The red blood corpuscles are nucleated, unlike those of mammals.

The lymphatic system

The lymphatic system in fowls also follows the same general pattern as in mammals. However, there are no lymph nodes but the bursa of Fabricius is present, which has no counterpart in mammals.

The endocrine system

This is fairly similar to that of mammals.

The nervous system

The nervous system corresponds to the mammalian system.

The spinal cord extends to the 3rd coccygeal vertebra. Derived from the spinal cord are the spinal nerves, which on each side number 15 cervical, 7 thoracic, 14 lumbo-sacral and a few coccygeal. Lying in the mid-line of the carcass just under the vertebrae are the *brachial* and *lumbo-sacral plexuses*. These are networks of nerves.

The brachial plexus consists of the last three cervical and the first two thoracic nerves.

The lumbo-sacral plexus consists of the last lumbar and the first four sacral nerves. This plexus can be exposed by removing the kidneys.

The *autonomic nervous system* is that part that regulates the activities of the viscera, including the heart. It is composed of the *sympathetic* and *parasympathetic* nerves, which have opposing effects. The sympathetic system consists of two chains of interconnected ganglia with connections to the spinal nerves.

The eye

The eye is relatively much larger than in mammals and has a much larger accurate field of vision. A structure within the eye that does not occur in mammals is the *pecten*. It is a black vertical comb or fan that overlies the optic nerve.

The lower eyelid is better developed than the upper. The third eyelid or *nictitating membrane* is extensive and capable of covering the complete anterior surface of the eye.

The ear

The external opening is small and covered with coarse feathers. There is no external auricle or ear flap.

The urogenital system

The *kidneys* (Fig. 23.12) are elongated, about 5 cm in length, three-lobed, brown in colour and soft in consistency. They lie in deep recesses in the pelvic bones formed by the last thoracic ribs and the 1st lumbar ribs to the 6th caudal vetebra. They almost fill the renal fossae. In front they are in contact with the lungs. The ureters emerge from the medial aspects of the middle lobes and enter the middle part of the cloaca – the urodeum. There is no bladder in the fowl. The product of the kidneys is not fluid like mammalian urine but is a semi-solid substance composed of urates. It shows up white in the droppings. As the consistency of the kidneys is soft it is difficult to remove them from the bony recesses without tearing.

The *testes* are ovoid, cream-coloured bodies. They lie just anterior to the kidneys and vary greatly in size according to age. During the breeding season they are greatly enlarged. The *deferent ducts* are convoluted and run parallel to and medial to the ureters. They enter the urodeal cavity of the cloaca. The straight terminal ends of the deferent ducts are muscular and act as ejaculatory ducts. There is no penis.

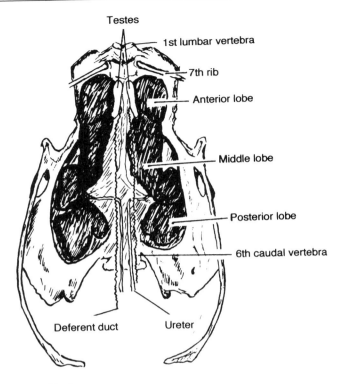

Fig. 23.12 Kidneys of fowl.

The *ovary* (Fig. 23.13) lies ventral to the left kidney. Only the left ovary is functional. The right one regresses soon after hatching. The ovary consists of a mass of spherical ova, which vary greatly in size during the laying season. The smallest ova are white in colour but as they increase in size they gradually become yellow. Mature ova measure 2–3 cm in diameter.

The *oviduct* consists of five parts, the divisions of which are not discernible to the naked eye:

(1) The *infandibulum* is about 10 cm in length and collects the ova from the ovary. The ova take about 18 minutes to pass through this part.

(2) The *magnum* is the largest part of the oviduct and measures about 35 cm in length. In this part the *albumen* or 'white of egg' is secreted. Passage through the magnum takes 3 hours.

(3) The *isthmus* is about 10 cm long. It produces the shell membranes. Passage through the isthmus takes $1\frac{1}{4}$ hours.

(4) The *uterus* or shell gland is about 10 cm long. It produces the hard shell. Passage through the uterus takes 20 hours.

(5) The *vagina* is about 8 cm long. It conveys the fully formed egg into the urodeal part of the cloaca to be expelled through the proctodeum and vent.

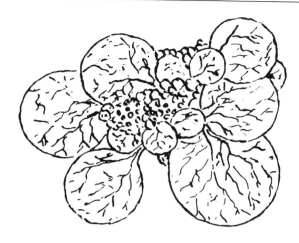

Fig. 23.13 Ovary of fowl.

Passage through the oviduct takes 24 hours and eggs may be laid either end first. If the shell is pigmented, the pigment is laid down during the last five hours in the oviduct.

The right oviduct is vestigial and is often represented by a transparent rudimentary tube.

The egg (Fig. 23.14)

The egg shell, although strong and rigid, is porous. Part of its strength is due to its curved shape.

The outer shell is composed of three layers, a middle *calcareous layer*, an outer *cuticle* and an inner *mammillary layer*. Inside the outer shell is the *shell mem-*

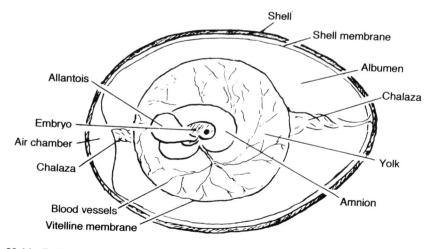

Fig. 23.14 Fertile egg.

brane, which consists of two layers. These two layers are separated at the larger end of the egg to form the *air chamber*. Contained in the shell membrane is the *albumen* or 'white of egg'. The albumen is composed of three layers: a thick layer in the middle surrounded by an outer and inner layer of thin watery albumen. At each end of the egg there is a denser twisted cord of albumen, the *chalaza*. The chalazae are attached to the yolk and keep it in place.

In the albumen is the yellow *yolk* of the egg. This consists of two types of cells, smaller white yolk cells and larger yellow yolk cells. The colour of the yolk depends upon the amount of xanthophyll in the diet. The yok is surrounded by the thin *vitelline membrane*.

Fertilised fowl eggs hatch 21 days after laying, turkey and duck eggs in 28 days and geeze in 30–35 days.

Unfertilised eggs of course have no embryos.

Chapter 24
Slaughter and Dressing of Poultry

Legislation provides for the humane slaughter and humane pre-slaughter treatment of poultry. It requires that

> no turkey, domestic fowl, guinea fowl, duck or goose shall be slaughtered unless it is slaughtered instantaneously by means of decapitation or dislocation of the neck or some other method approved by the Ministers, or it is, by stunning affected by means of an instrument of a kind approved by them and in proper repair, instantaneously rendered insensible to pain until death supervenes.

The Jewish and Muslim methods, i.e. ritual, are exempt in the legislation.

The majority of birds are killed and dressed at poultry packing stations. The following is a typical process.

Unloading bay

The transport vehicles reverse into the bay, which is under cover. The birds, which are carried either in fixed or loose plastic crates, are unloaded and individually hung upside down by the feet on to shackles suspended from a continuously moving line. The centres of the shackles are approximately 15 cm apart. Such a line can have a throughput of up to 8000 birds per hour or 135 birds per minute. Ante-mortem inspection is carried out in this area. Crates are provided for birds rejected by the inspector. These are dealt with separately.

Slaughter room

The birds enter the slaughter room through a small narrow opening and are stunned instantaneously. Before stunning a quietening time is allowed, i.e. the time between hanging and stunning, of not more than 6 minutes for turkeys and not more than 3 minutes for domestic fowls.

Various types of electrical stunners are used. The birds are stunned either by their heads coming into contact with a 500-volt electrified metal slope or wires. In the most common type, the birds' heads pass through a 150-volt electrically charged water bath.

Recent research by various workers has shown that it is more humane to kill the birds in the stunner than just to stun them. Bleeding is not affected in any way.

Bleeding
About 30 seconds after passing through the stunners the birds are bled auto-matically or by an operator who severs either the right or left jugular vein at the base of the skull. The birds now pass along a bleeding tunnel for at least 2 minutes for turkeys and at least 90 seconds for domestic fowls. This is to allow the birds to bleed before entering the scalding process. It is estimated that 50% of the blood is removed.

Scalding
The birds, still suspended from the line, pass through the scald tank in which there is continuously changing water at 50–80°C, usually 53°C (soft scald) or 63°C (hard scald). The time in the scald should be no more than 2 minutes. This ensures that the skin will be untorn and unblemished. Higher times and tem-peratures result in torn and discoloured skins. The scalding loosens the feathers for the defeathering process. Sometimes detergents are added to the scald water. This helps in penetration of the water to the feather follicles.

Defeathering
The birds pass into the defeathering machines, which consist of revolving drums with rubber beaters or discs. The birds are continually flailed or scraped by these, while being sprayed with warm water. This process takes approximately 1 min-ute. Any feathers still remaining attached are removed by hand. Ducks are often further defeathered by a hot wax process which removes the finer feathers and down.

   The first post-mortem inspection takes place in this area. Rejected birds are removed from the line.

   After plucking, the birds are washed by overhead sprays.

Neck slitting and foot removal
A vertical incision is made in the skin on the dorsal surface of the neck to assist in the removal of the crop, oesophagus and trachea at a later stage. The feet are removed automatically by a cutter on the line or by manually operated secateurs. The birds drop on to a conveyor that transfers them through a narrow opening from the 'dirty' section of the slaughterhouse into the 'clean' section.

Evisceration line
The birds are rehung by the hocks on to the shackles of the evisceration line. The line is continuous from this transfer point right through to the washing and cooling tanks. The evisceration line runs above a water trough or a mechanical conveyor, which carries away waste materials. Various operations are carried out on this line:

(1)   *Venting*. This is done by using a venting gun or scissors. In either method the vent is cut round so that it can be removed with the intestines from the

carcass. Great care is needed in this important operation if faecal contamination of the carcass, edible offals and operators' hands is to be avoided.

(2) *Drawing.* All of the viscera are drawn out of the body cavity, leaving them hanging from the carcass ready for inspection. The drawing is done either by hand or by operators using eviscerating forks or by automatic eviscerating machines.

At this point the inspectors examine the viscera, the body cavity and the carcass generally. Good lighting, properly directed into the body cavity, is essential.

(3) *Removal of offals.* The edible offals or giblets, i.e. the heart, liver and gizzard, are removed for further cleaning aand washing. The intestines, proventriculus and lungs are discarded into the water trough or mechanical conveyor. On some lines a suction tube is then introduced into the body cavity to remove any contamination or portions of lungs remaining.

(4) *Head removal.* Various techniques are used by the heads are generally removed mechanically by traction of a head puller on the line. This also removes the crop, oesophagus and trachea. An inspector or a quality control officer then examines the carcass generally, especially the body cavity.

(5) *Neck removal.* The necks are removed by cutting through the vertebrae between the shoulders using automatic or manual secateurs. The necks are classified as part of the edible offal or giblets.

(6) *Line washing.* Before going into the washing and cooling tanks the birds are spray washed to remove blood and extraneous matter.

(7) *Polyphosphate injection.* When polyphosphates are used they are injected under pressure by guns with two hollow perforated needles. The solution is injected into the breast and sometimes also into the leg muscles. Up to 5% of the body weight of this permitted additive solution may be injected.

Washing

The birds are dropped automatically from the evisceration line into long spin washer tanks, which contain mains water at a temperature of 10–16°C. The birds enter at a body temperature of 36°C, remain in the washer for about 10 minutes and leave the washer at about 24°C, a reduction of 11°C. The birds are propelled along the tanks by revolving paddes. The water through the tanks may be with or against (contra-flow) the direction of the birds. Chlorination is used at a level of 50 ppm free chlorine, which almost completely kills bacteria in the tanks.

Chilling

The birds are transferred from the washer unit by an elevator into the long immersion chiller tank. This works on the same principle as the washer unit. Flake ice is dropped into the water in the chiller tank from overhead flake-ice machines. Some chillers are fed with refrigerated water. The birds remain in the chiller tank for 30–40 minutes and leave at a temperature of 2–4°C.

Draining

After chilling, the birds are hung by the hocks on an overhead conveyor or draining line for 10 minutes to lose any surplus water not sealed in or absorbed by the skin or muscle during washing and chilling.

Freezing

After draining, the birds are packed into polythene bags and frozen to a temperature of −18°C.

Fresh-chilled birds

Instead of freezing, some birds are sold for the fresh trade. They are chilled in air chillers or by CO_2 to a surface temperature of 0 to −1°C (super chilled). Their temperature must not exceed 4°C.

'New York dressed', or 'not yet dressed' (NYD) poultry or 'long-legged' poultry, are birds that have been defeathered and chilled. They are sold uneviscerated and with the feet and head left on the carcass. Inspection therefore cannot be very thorough.

Inspection of poultry

Where the line system of killing and dressing of poultry is in operation the inspection is divided as follows.

(1)   Ante-mortem inspection
(2)   Post-mortem:

    (a)   whole carcass inspection
    (b)   evisceration inspection
    (c)   final carcass inspection.

NB   At all inspection points the lighting must be good and well directed (540 lux).

Ante-mortem inspection

When this has been carried out as a flock inspection at the place of origin by an official veterinary officer and within 24 hours of arrival at the slaughterhouse, only a further general check is necessary. If not, each bird is inspected on the line in the unloading bay. Adequate lighting is essential and at leat 2 metres of line is required for the inspector. Crates should be provided for birds rejected by the inspector, and containers for birds dead on arrival.

Post-mortem inspection

(1)   Whole carcass inspection is carried out immediately after defeathering and before any other operation. Badly bled or emaciated birds, and birds with

septic wounds, etc. are taken off the line before they can pass through into the 'clean' section of the slaughterhouse.

(2) Evisceration inspection. One inspector should be able to inspect 1200 broiler fowls per hour provided the health level of the birds is good. If a batch of birds shows a high incidence of disease, the line should be slowed down accordingly. Twelve hundred broilers are equivalent to 600 hens or 900 ducks or 600 turkeys, which are more difficult to inspect. In hens the larger ova are the first things to be taken out of the body cavity. Whole eggs are expressed out through the cloaca. These must remain identifiable with the carcass. Care has to be taken so that they are not broken. In ducks the livers are friable so more care has to be taken in removing the viscera. The partly eviscerated birds are inspected still with the viscera attached. This includes the intestines, gizzard, liver, spleen, heart, lungs and the ovary in hens. There are various techniques of inspection but within the very limited time available for inspection of each bird, the viscera, body cavity (including the forward air sacs), legs and carcass must be examined.

(3) Final carcass inspection. This takes place after the viscera have been removed and the body cavity has been washed. This may be done by a quality control officer.

At the inspection points on the line there must be lighting of a proper intensity (540 lux) and properly directed. There must also be warm-water hand sprays, wash-hand basins and knife sterilisers at appropriate points. It is important that good hygiene be maintained throughout the slaughterhouse regarding floors, walls, ceilings, plant, operators and operators' clothes.

Chapter 25
Diseases of Poultry

The diseases have been listed in alphabetical order for ease of reference. Where diseases have more than one name, the commonest name is given first. It is suggested that, in conjunction with this section, the reader refers to a suitable textbook showing coloured illustrations of the various poultry diseases since many of these diseases share similar lesions.

Abscesses

In poultry, abscesses tend not to have thick capsules. The contained pus is often dry and odourless. They occur secondarily to such conditions as breast blisters, treading wounds and cannibalism wounds.

Judgement: Local trimming may be sufficient.

Aflatoxicosis

See under *Penicillium* on p. 166.

Judgement: Total rejection.

Air sacculitis

Poultry reared in broiler houses are the most susceptible, and large percentages may be affected. It is caused by *Mycoplasma gallisepticum* or *M. synoviae*, very often in association with *Escherichia coli*. The thin walls of the air sacs, instead of being clear, glistening and transparent, become cloudy, opaque and yellow. Later the sacs become filled with a thick white or yellow pus. The condition often progresses to an *E. coli* septicaemia.

Judgement: Total rejection.

Ascites or dropsy

This is the accumulation of an excess of fluid in the body cavity. It is most obvious in the vent region when the bird is suspended by the head or neck [Plate 7(b)]. The ascitic fluid may be present in great quantity. It is most often associated with disease of the viscera, especially the liver, and with tumours. Putrefaction – the green colour that is first seen around the vent – rapidly ensues.

Judgement: Total rejection.

Aspergillosis

The causal organism of this poultry disease is *Aspergillus fumigatus*. Infection is by inhalation of the spores of the fungus, which is widely distributed in nature, e.g. in hay, straw and litter. The symptoms in young birds are generally those of an acute respiratory disease, i.e. difficult breathing, gasping and sneezing. There is loss of appetite, thirst, diarrhoea and emaciation. The post-mortem lesions are found most often in the lungs. These consist of greyish white or yellow caseous nodules varying in size from a pin head up to a small pea. Similar nodules occur also in the air sacs and body cavity. The commonest lesions in adult fowls are large, firm, decaying masses, yellow in colour, in the air sacs, which may be lined by a greenish black, fur-like growth of mould. Ducks as well as turkeys are commonly affected.

Judgement: Total rejection.

Avian leukosis complex

The complex consists of three virus diseases although there are other groupings: (1) lymphoid leukosis, (2) myeloid leukosis, and (3) erythroid leukosis (erythroblastosis).

Marek's disease is sometimes included.

Lymphoid leukosis

This is the most important. It is difficult to differentiate macroscopically from Marek's disease except in certain specific cases.

The first lesions occur as small nodular lymphoid tumours, which cannot always be seen by the naked eye in the bursa of Fabricius. These are smooth, glistening and soft and on cross-section are creamy white to grey. Secondary tumours can occur in any organ but are most common in the liver. They may have a nodular or diffuse distribution. When the liver is diffusely affected, it is usually very large and extends the full length of the body cavity ('big liver disease') [Plate 8(d)].

Judgement: Total rejection.

Myeloid leukosis

The liver has a morocco-leather-like appearance. Nodular discrete tumours, which have a chalky consistency, may also occur in the spleen and kidneys and on the inside of the body cavity walls.

Judgement: Total rejection.

Erythroid leukosis (erythroblastosis)
This is a rare disease in which the liver is enlarged and cherry red in colour as also are the spleen and bone marrow.
   Judgement: Total rejection.

Bacillary white diarrhoea (BWD)

See pullorum disease on p. 272.

Blackhead *(infectious entero-hepatitis or histomoniasis)*

This is a specific infectious disease chiefly of turkeys but which may also affect chickens and pheasants. It is caused by the protozoan parasite *Histomonas meleagridis*. This is commonly spread by the caecal worm *Heterakis gallinarum*. Direct infection through the faeces may occur.
   Affected birds lose their appetite, and exhibit dullness, weakness, and drooping wings and tails. These symptoms, however, are common to many poultry diseases. In turkeys there are characteristic yellow droppings. In the acute form, death is rapid but a chronic wasting may be seen in older birds. Cyanosis or blackening of the wattles and skin of the head may appear, hence the name blackhead. However, this is by no means a constant feature nor is it confined to this diease. The characteristic lesions, although they are secondary to caecal lesions, are found in the liver. They consist of circular areas of focal necrosis up to 1 cm in diameter. They are depressed and yellow to yellowish green with greyish peripheral regions. Coalescing may occur to form large areas of necrosis. They may extend deeply into the liver, which is enlarged. The early lesions in the caeca are small haemorrhagic ulcers. Later one or both caecal tubes may be greatly enlarged with thickened walls and containing dark cheesy masses.
   Judgement: Dependent upon the severity of the lesions.

Breast blisters

These are common and as the name suggests are blisters that occur in the skin of the breast over the keel of the sternum. They are due to injury and most are caused by pressure, while resting, on the breast bone. A false bursa develops that contains serous fluid. This may become infected with the formation of a large abscess, which can extend into the breast muscles and even into the bony sternum [Plate 7(a)]. Breast blisters, as well as sore hocks, are common in birds with diseases of the feet or joints, e.g. bumblefoot and synovitis.
   Judgement: Trimming of the affected part may be all that is necessary but where muscle and bone are affected the whole carcass should be rejected.

Bruising

This can occur during catching, crating, transporting and uncrating of birds. It may be the result of shackling of the legs on the line before slaughter. The most common place to find bruising is on the legs and on the body at the hip joints. Bruising may be very extensive because of under-running of the skin, which is loosely attached in the fowl. It may be highly coloured, blue, green and red colours predominating. It is important not to confuse bruises with putrefaction as the colours can be very similar [Plate 8(a)].

Judgement: Dependent upon the extent and severity of the lesions.

Bumblefoot

This is a non-infectious, localised, bulbous lesion of the ball of the foot and is commonly seen in domestic fowls. It is thought to be due either to a foreign body penetrating the foot or to bruising. Abscesses may occur due to a secondary infection. It is closely associated with plantar necrosis.

Judgement: Local trimming.

Cannibalism

Birds kept in overcrowded conditions are liable to cannibalism. It is part of the 'pecking order' and is a form of bullying. Boredom is also a factor. Fluorescent lighting, installed without fitted red filters, is thought to have been the cause in some cases. Birds peck at other birds' heads, backs, wings and vents causing wounds. In mild cases the skin is discoloured but in severe cases extensive wounds occur and death can result. As a preventative measure birds are often debeaked; i.e. they have about one-third trimmed off the upper beak [Plate 8(b)].

Judgement: Dependent upon the severity of the lesions.

Coccidiosis

Coccidiosis in poultry is caused by *Eimeria* species. Six of these are considered to be pathogenic to poultry, and it is convenient to group them according to the parts of the intestine that they affect.

Eimeria acervulina and *E. praecox* affect mainly the duodenum. *Eimeria acervulina* may cause a severe disease with lesions varying from petechial hae-morrhages to severe haemorrhage of the duodenal musosa. *Eimeria praecox* causes only a mild infection.

Eimeria necatrix, *E. maxima* and *E. brunetti* affect the middle part of the small intestine. *Eimeria maxima* causes similar lesions. *Eimeria brunetti* causes hae-morrhagic lesions generally in the terminal part of the small intestine.

Eimeria tenella causes characteristic haemorrhages and white spots in the caeca, which are often filled with coagulated blood and necrotic material.

Judgement: Dependent upon the state of the carcass, which is often emaciated and oedematous.

Coli-granuloma (Hjärre's disease)

Granulomatous lesions caused by *E. coli* are found mainly in the wall of the caeca but also in the rest of the intestine and the liver.

Judgement: Dependent upon the state of the carcass.

Curled toe syndrome (curled toe paralysis)

In this condition the toes are turned in owing to the paralysis. It is thought to be due to deficiency of vitamin B_2.

Judgement: Dependent upon the state of the carcass.

Egg peritonitis

Affected birds are almost always in good body condition and are generally fat with a prominent abdomen. All the viscera are covered by a yellow yolk-like material, which comes from the bird's own reproductive system. Obviously male birds are not affected. The oviduct is usually impacted with solidified 'yolk', and egg yolks of varying size are found lying free in the body cavity. Egg binding may also be found, i.e. when a fully formed egg becomes impacted in the oviduct.

Judgement: Total rejection.

Emaciation

This is a common cause of rejection of poultry and is generally associated with a chronic disease. The muscles are wasted and flabby and there is an absence of fat.

Judgement: Total rejection.

Erysipelas

The causal organism is *Erysipelothrix rhusiopathiae (insidiosa)*. Turkeys are most commonly affected but it also occurs in domestic fowls. In the acute form it is septicaemic in type with haemorrhages in the skin, particularly of the head, heart and breast muscles. The liver and spleen may be enlarged with fibrinous deposits. The lungs are often brown in colour instead of the normal bright red.

The chronic form is characterised by thickening and black discoloration of the skin of the head hence the name 'leatherhead'. There may be an endocarditis and an arthritis with a purulent synovitis.

Care should be taken in handling birds affected or erysipeloid may be contracted.

Judgement: Total rejection.

Escherichia (E.) coli septicaemia

This occurs mainly in broilers and is generally triggered off by a mycoplasma infection and or an infectious bronchitis virus infection followed by the *E. coli* infection.

It is without doubt the most frequent cause of rejection of poultry. A large percentage of birds from a broiler house, which may contain up to 20 000 birds, can be affected. When such a batch of birds is slaughtered, inspection on the line becomes a serious problem, necessitating a slowing down of the line.

The organs in the body cavity, especially the heart and the liver, become coated with a fibrino-purulent exudate. This may be thick, yellow and gelatinous or thin, white and inspissated. The birds are often emaciated. The condition is often associated with an air sacculitis [Plate 8(c)].

Judgement: Total rejection.

Fat necrosis

Fat necrosis is uncommon in birds. It occurs generally in very fat birds in the fat of the body cavity. The affected fat is denser in consistency and has a dull greyish appearance.

Judgement: Local trimming.

Fatty liver syndrome

This occurs in very fat laying hens, usually during spells of hot weather. The liver is generally enlarged, friable and of a yellow colour similar to the body fat. It is greasy to the touch. The body fat may be very soft and almost of a liquid consistency. Death due to liver haemorrhage may follow.

Judgement: Dependent upon the state of the carcass. Reject liver.

Fowl paralysis

See Marek's disease on p. 270.

Fowl pest

Fowl pest, including Newcastle disease and fowl plague, is a notifiable disease.

Newcastle disease
This is a fatal virus disease that spreads rapidly through a flock. Clinically

affected birds have a high temperature and adopt a very sleepy attitude but drink freely. Respirations may be characteristic with long gasping inhalations. A frothy exudate may hang from the beak. At post-mortem, haemorrhages of the pre-ventriculus are present and haemorrhages and ulceration of the intestine are common lesions.

Imported captive birds, especially of the parrot family, have been found to have been infected. Recent outbreaks in poultry have been traced to poultry food contaminated by feral pigeons' faeces containing paramyxovirus.

Upon confirmation of the disease all birds in the infected flock are slaughtered immediately and a restriction upon the movements of poultry and hatching eggs is imposed in the surrounding area until the disease is eradicated.

Newcastle disease virus causes an influenza-like disease in humans.

Judgement: Total rejection.

Fowl plague

This is a rare disease caused by a virus. Although it is grouped with Newcastle disease, it is entirely different. The clinical symptoms and post-mortem findings are very similar. The two diseases can only be differentiated by isolation of the viruses.

Judgement: Total rejection.

Fowl pox

Domestic fowls, turkeys and pigeons are affected by this virus disease. It is characterised by dry or moist wart-like growths on the unfeathered parts parti-cularly of the head, i.e. face, eyelids, cere, comb and wattles, and of the legs and feet. The warts are raised, hard, firmly attached, nodular-rounded scabs, brownish in colour. Dull, pale yellow, firmly attached plaques of solidified pus in the form of diphtheritic membranes occur in the mouth and pharynx.

The symptoms are loss of appetite, dullness, infertility, discharge from the eyes and nostrils and a diphtheritic membrane in the mouth that may cause suffoca-tion.

Judgement: Total rejection.

Fowl typhoid

This is a serious septicaemic disease of domestic fowls, and is one that can also occur in turkeys. The causal organism is *Salmonella gallinarum*. In acute cases death occurs quickly after infection. The carcass has a jaundiced appearance and there is congestion and enlargement of the liver and spleen. The liver has a typical bronzed appearance and the lungs are brown in colour. There may be degeneration of the ovary.

Judgement: Total rejection.

Freezer burn

This is caused by over-or prolonged refrigeration of carcasses. The lesions are due to local surface desiccation. They show as abnormal coloured patches on the skin. They vary from white and yellow to dark brown [Plate 7(c)].

Judgement: Dependent upon the severity of the condition.

Gangrenous dermatitis

This is a disease of poultry caused by *Staphylococcus aureus* and *Clostridium perfringens*. Evil-smelling lesions occur anywhere on the skin but mainly on the breast and vent region.

Judgement: Total rejection.

Gapes

This is caused by the roundworm, *Syngamus trachea*, which occurs in the trachea of fowl and turkey. The worms are red in colour and the males and females are found permanently attached in copulation. The male is very much smaller than the female, measuring 2–6 mm, and is attached to the anterior third of the female, which measures up to 2 cm in length. The eggs, which are produced in the trachea, are coughed up, swallowed by the host and passed out in the faeces. They reach the infective stage in about 3 days. Infection may be direct by fowl swallowing the infective eggs or larvae or indirect by eaging earthworms, snails or slugs containing infective larvae. The larvae penetrate the intestinal wall of the fowl and are carried by the bloodstream to the lungs. The young worms migrate to the large bronchi and then to the trachea where they attach themselves to the mucous membrane and suck blood, hence their red colour. Heavy infestations may cause pneumonia and catarrhal tracheitis. Young birds are most often affected and the characteristic signs of the disease, which is known as gapes, are the gaping extended beak and the spasmodic gasping for breath. In laying birds egg production is reduced. Occasionally birds die from asphyxia.

Judgement: Emaciated carcasses are rejected.

Gout

This is the deposition of salt of uric acid. It is found most commonly in the joints of the feet and legs but may also be found on the surface of the heart and liver when it is known as visceral gout. The depositions are found as accumulations of a white, dry and non-purulent material.

Judgement: Local rejection when joints are affected. Total rejection in visceral gout.

Gumboro disease (infectious bursal disease)

The disease is caused by a virus and is highly infectious with a high mortality. It affects domestic fowls mainly from 3 to 6 weeks of age. The bursa of Fabricius becomes enlarged and inflamed. As this is the site of formation of antibodies the immune system is affected. Birds that recover have therefore a lower resistance to many diseases, especially gangrenous dermatitis. A common finding is an inspissated abscess in the bursa.

Judgement: Total rejection.

Hernia or rupture

This is found generally as a loop of bowel, just under the skin, which has passed through a tear in the abdominal muscles.

Judgement: Local trimming.

Hexamitiasis

Young turkeys are affected by the protozoan parasite *Hexamita meleagridis*, which causes a catarrhal enteritis.

Judgement: Dependent upon the state of the carcass.

Histamoniasis

See blackhead on p. 263.

Infectious bronchitis

See gapes on p. 268.

Infectious bursal disease

See Gumboro disease above.

Infectious sinusitis

The causal organism is a mycoplasma. Turkeys are most often affected, showing pronounced swelling of the infra-orbital sinuses, which become filled with a thick, yellow exudate.

Judgement: Rejection of the head is usually sufficient.

Jaundice

This is not common in poultry. When it does occur it is generally in association with liver damage. The Rimmington and Fowrie test (p. 105) is useful for diagnosis.

Judgement: Total rejection.

Keratoconjunctivitis

Insanitary conditions, with the production of ammonia, are the cause of the condition, which is characterised by inflammation and swelling of the eyelids, and scab formation with the closure of the eyes. In severe cases ulceration of the cornea occurs. As a result of birds rubbing their eyes, the feathers of the shoulders are often dirty and matted. Fowls and turkeys are affected.

Judgement: Dependent upon the state of the carcass.

Kinky back

See spondylolisthesis on p. 275.

Lice

See p. 162.

Machine damage

Various types of damage are caused by the machinery at poultry slaughterhouses. If the damage is done before slaughter, bruising due to bleeding takes place. Legs or wings can be bruised or fractured during shackling in the unloading bay. In damage after death there is no bleeding as the blood circulation has stopped. Most machine damage occurs in the defeathering machine where the skin can be torn and legs or wings broken or dislocated. When the skin is torn, contamination of the underlying muscles takes place and pockets of water can be trapped under the skin.

Judgement: Dependent upon the degree of damage.

Marble spleen disease (lung oedema)

This is a virus disease of pheasants. The main lesions are seen in the spleen, which is enlarged and mottled giving a marbling effect. The lungs are often oedematous.

Judgement: Total rejection.

Marek's disease (fowl paralysis)

This is a virus disease of fowls that, except in certain specific cases, is not distinguishable macroscopically from lymphoid leukosis. In a typical case where the brachial and sciatic nerves are affected, partial or complete paralysis of the wings and legs occurs, hence the name 'fowl paralysis'. Affected nerves are enlarged with a change in colour from white to grey or yellow.

The acute form may cause death with few or no symptoms, the post-mortem lesions being small lymphoid tumours in the viscera, skin and muscles.

In the chronic form the lymphoid tumours are larger, pale and circumscribed and are indistinguishable macroscopically from those of lymphoid leukosis. Microscopically the cellular structure is different. There is diffuse enlargement of the bursa of Fabricius or of the thymus. The lesions in the muscles (breast muscles in particular) and in the skin are most noticeable when the bird has been defeathered. The skin tumours are associated with the feather follicles.

Skin, muscles and nerves are not affected in lymphoid leukosis.

Most birds are vaccinated against Marek's disease with a very efficient vaccine. *Judgement:* Total rejection.

Moulds

The moulds described for red meats on pages 165 and 166 will also affect poultry in the same way. Plate 7(d) shows *Cladosporium herbarum* infection of a turkey.

Newcastle disease

See fowl pest on p. 266.

Oregon disease *(degenerative myopathy)*

This disease of turkeys and poultry is considered to be hereditary in origin. Alternatively it may be due to rough handling of the wings while restraining for injections, etc. The condition only affects the deep portion of the breast muscle, the so-called 'fillet muscle'. It can be either uni-or bilateral and is caused by inadequate blood supply to the affected muscle.

In the early stages affected muscle shows an area of reddish to green coloration, which later changes to yellow, dark green and dark brown. The colour changes are probably due to breakdown pigments of haemoglobin or myoglobin.

In the final stages there is atrophy of the fillet muscle or muscles, showing in the breast as an identation or indentations if the condition is bilateral [Plate 8(e)]. *Judgement:* Remove affected parts.

Osteopetrosis (Paget's disease, thick leg disease or marble bone)

This is often included in the avian leukosis complex. It is a rare condition characterised by gross thickening of the bones, particularly the long bones of the leg. Joints are not affected and the bones of the feet seldom.

Externally the bones lose their smooth surfaces and become rough and pitted.

Internally the medullary cavities are greatly reduced in size and the bones become enlarged, heavy, extremely hard and difficult to break.

Judgement: Total rejection.

Perosis (slipped tendon)

Manganese deficiency is the cause of this condition, which occurs in chickens and turkey poults. The tibi-metatarsal joints become enlarged and deformed. Because of the malformation the gastrocnemius tendons slip out of the condyles to either the inner or outer sides. This causes the 'bow legged' or 'knock-kneed' appearance. One or both legs may be affected. The keel of the sternum is often bent. Affected birds are often in poor condition because of their inability to reach their food.

Judgement: Trim unless emaciated.

Plantar necrosis

There is necrosis and exfoliation of the skin on the ball of the foot. It is probably due to caking of faecal material on the foot. This causes an accumulation of dead tissue and provides a suitable site for the growth of bacteria. It is closely associated with bumble foot.

Judgement: Local rejection.

Prolapse

Protrusion of part of the bowel and/or cloaca through the vent is common in poultry. A common cause is breakage of an egg in the oviduct or cloaca causing straining. The condition may be caused by or be the cause of cannibalism.

Judgement: Trim.

Pullorum disease (bacillary white diarrhoea, BWD)

The causal agent is *Salmonella pullorum*. In the adult form the liver is enlarged with multiple necrotic foci and a fibrinous exudate; the heart is enlarged and deformed; and the kidneys are enlarged.

The chronic form is characterised by an acute or chronic pericarditis and the ova are discoloured, shrunken and sometimes cystic.

Judgement: Total rejection.

Pustular typhilitis

This is characterised by numerous, round, hard, lumpy swellings affecting the caeca. The lymphoid patches at their entrance, the so-called caecal tonsils, are often enlarged to the size of a hazel nut. Other similar swellings occur at intervals along the caecal walls. Cross-sections of the swellings show firm outer walls with caseous centres. Rarely there are similar lesions in the liver.

The cause is unknown but it is thought to be secondary to parasitic damage.

Judgement: Total rejection.

Putrefaction

As staleness develops in the carcass, the eyes become opaque and sunk in their sockets. The feet are hard and stiff and the muscles loose, flabby and darker in colour. An unpleasant odour develops and a green colour appears, especially in the regions of the vent and crop. It is important not to confuse the colour of putrefaction with that of bruising.

Judgement: Total rejection.

Red mite (Dermanyssus gallinae)

Dermanyssus gallinae (Fig. 25.1) is the common mite of the domestic fowl and turkey. It is white to red in colour and visible to the naked eye. It is nocturnal in habit and feeds (sucking blood) on the birds at night, whilst living in cracks and crevices during the day. After feeding, the mites are bright red and much more easily seen. Heavy infestations may cause an anaemia.

The mite may cause irritation to humans and other animals, particularly horses.

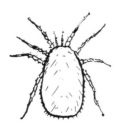

Fig. 25.1 *Dermanyssus gallinae* (× 30).

Rickets (vitamin D deficiency)

Deformities of the bones occur which arae most evident in the legs. The joints become enlarged. The ribs show the typical 'beading' and the keel of the sternum is often bent. The beak, bones and claws are soft and pliable.

Judgement: Total rejection.

Round heart disease

Turkeys are mainly affected but occasionally chickens also. The cause is unknown. The heart is enlarged and distorted so that the apex becomes very

much rounded instead of pointed. The liver is also enlarged with rounded edges.
Judgement: Dependent upon the state of the carcass.

Roundworms

(1) *Ascaridia galli* and *A. dissimilis* occur in chickens and turkeys, respectively. Unless they occur in large numbers they are not important. They are found in the small intestines and the male worms are about half the size of the females, which measure about 6 cm × 1 mm. The eggs are passed in the faeces and reach the infective stage in about 2 weeks. The eggs when swallowed develop in the small intestine. Heavy infestations cause a hae-morrhagic enteritis and may even lead to complete obstruction of the intestine.

A condition called 'spotty liver syndrome' has been found in poultry with heavy ascarid infection (cf. 'milk spot liver' in pigs). The livers had multiple white lesions up to 2 mm in diameter, but whether these were due to the ascarid infection is not known.

(2) *Syngamus trachea* (see gapes, p. 268).
(3) *Heterakis gallinarum* occurs in the caeca of turkeys and fowls and measures 7–15 mm in length. It is important because it is a carrier of *Histomonas meleagridis*, which causes blackhead.
(4) *Capillaria.* Several species of these thread-or hairworms are found in poultry. *Capillaria obsignata* and *C. caudinflata* cause an enteritis by bur-rowing into the mucosa of the small intestine; *C. annaulata* and *C. contorta* are found in the mucosa of the oesophagus and crop.

Judgement: Dependent upon the state of the carcass.

Ruptured gastrocnemius tendons

The tendons are usually completely ruptured with accompanying haemorrhage. Occasionally the condition is unilateral. The cause is unknown.
Judgement: Trim.

Salmonella diseases

Various diseases are caused by *Salmonella* species.

(1) *Salmonella pullorum* (see pullorum disease, p. 272).
(2) *Salmonella galinarum* (see fowl typhoid, p. 267).
(3) *Salmonella typhimurium* and *S. enteritidis* can cause severe diseases in poultry that are indistinguishable from pullorum disease. These two salmonellae are commonly associated with food poisoning in man and it is particularly important that duck eggs should be boiled for at least 10

minutes before eating. When flocks are found to be infected with *S. enteritidis* or *S. typhimurium*, they are slaughtered.

(4)   *Salmonella virchow* has also been associated with poultry meat causing food poisoning.
     Judgement: Total rejection.

Salpingitis

This is inflammation of the oviduct probably caused by *E. coli*. The oviduct is inflammatory or impacted with a yellow exudate. Chickens or hens may be infected. It is fairly common in ducks.
     Judgement: Trim.

Scaly leg

The scaly leg mite *Cnemidocoptes mutans* burrows into the unfeathered parts of legs and feet causing proliferation and formation of coarse scales and crusts.
     Judgement: Trim affected parts.

Shovel beak or beak necrosis

This is caused by an accumulation of dry food inside the mouth along the edges of the beak. Necrosis and in severe cases sloughing of the beak occur.
     Judgement: Trim.

Spondylolisthesis (kinky back)

There appears to be a hereditary disposition to this type of paralysis in broiler fowls. The birds are unable to rise because of a complete or partial paralysis of the legs. The birds squat on their hocks. The paralysis occurs because of pressure on or rupture of the spinal cord due to malformation of the vertebrae in the thoracic region.
     Judgement: Dependent upon the state of the carcass.

Synovitis

Synovitis of the legs is common in poultry. The joints and tendon sheaths become swollen and filled with exudates. Many organisms are involved, e.g. staphylococci, *E. coli*, *Mycoplasma synoviae*, *Erysipelothrix rhusiopathiae* and viruses.
     Judgement: Dependent upon the severity of the condition, the organism involved and the state of the carcass.

Tapeworms (cestodes)

These are not important because with new methods of production birds lack contact with intermediate hosts, e..g. snails, beetles, ants and earthworms.

Three tapeworms affect poultry: *Davinia proglottina*, *Raillietina echinobothrida* and *R. tetragona*.

Thrush, moniliasis or candidiasis

This is an infectious disease of the crop of young turkeys (poults). The mortality rate is generally high. The causal organism is a fungus – *Candida albicans*. The crop is usually empty. The mucous membrane is slimy, thickened with whitish, circular, raised ulcers. The ulcers flake off leaving raw areas. Similar lesions occasionally occur in the mouth and oesophagus.

Judgement: Dependent upon the state of the carcass.

Tissue mite nodules

The tissue, subcutaneous or flesh mite *Laminosioptes cysticola* burrows through the skin and causes the formation of yellowish white, caseous and calcareous nodules about 2 mm in diameter in the subcutaneous tissue and most often on the surfaces of the breast muscles.

Judgement: Total rejection.

Tread wounds

Severe woulds may be caused on the back and sides of the body in the female during mating by the nails of the male. As a preventative measure 'toe cutting' is done in males within 3 days of hatching [Plate 8(f)].

Judgement: Dependent upon the extent of the wounds and whether sepsis is present.

Tuberculosis

This affects all species of birds and is caused by *Mycobacterium avium*. Present systems of rearing poultry have greatly reduced the incidence. Infected faeces are the mode of transmission to other birds and pigs. The lesions are typical yellowish white nodules or tubercles, which are found in the liver, spleen, intestines and occasionally in the lungs, bones and thymus. Lesions tend to coalesce to form larger nodules with smaller nodules on their surfaces. They shell out fairly easily from the liver and spleen and on cross-section are firm, and yellow with several small yellower foci. Calcification does not occur.

Judgement: Total rejection.

Tumours

The incidence of tumours in poultry is high. Lymphoid tumours are the commonest because of the prevalence of lymphoid lekosis and Marek's disease. The viscera are the common sites of tumours, especially the ovary and the liver. Ascites often ensues. Fibrous tumours are fairly common.

Judgement: Total rejection.

Turkey rhinotracheitis

This is a highly infectious disease of mainly young birds caused by a virus. There is inflammation of the upper respiratory tract, i.e. of the nasal passages, sinuses and the trachea. The main symptoms are nasal discharges, head shaking and difficulty in breathing, lack of appetite and emaciation.

Judgement: Total rejection.

Twisted-leg disease

The condition occurs in broilers from 2 to 6 weeks old. There is an outward twisting and bending of the condyles at the tibio-metatarsal joints. It is usually unilateral. The gastrocnemius tendons slip out of position. The resulting 'knock-kneed' deformity is very similar to that of perosis except that in twisted-leg disease there is no swelling of the joints. The cause is unknown.

Judgement: Dependent upon the state of the carcass.

Ulcerative enteritis (quail disease)

Oval or circular ulcers are found throughout the length of the intestinal mucosa. The contents of the intestine are often dark in colour. Small necrotic foci may occur in the liver. The disease is probably of bacterial origin.

Judgement: Total rejection.

Virus hepatitis of ducks

This is an acute and very infectious disease of young ducks. The typical lesions are petechial haemorrhages in the liver that persist in older birds.

Judgement: Total rejection.

Xanthomatosis

The skin, particularly of the breast, abdomen and legs, becomes yellow, thickened and rough. In the early stages there may be unilateral or bilateral swellings of the wattles.

Judgement: Total rejection.

Chapter 26
Affections of Specific Parts of Poultry

Affections of specific parts

NB   Tumours are common in poultry and can be found in many organs and tissues.

Body cavity

(1)   Air sacculitis (p. 261).
(2)   Aspergillosis (p. 262).
(3)   Egg peritonitis (p. 265).
(5)   Oedema (p. 100).
(6)   Myeloid leukosis (p. 262).

Bone

(1)   Breast blisters (p. 263).
(2)   Curled toe (p. 265).
(3)   Erythroid leukosis (p. 263).
(4)   Fractures (p. 270).
(5)   Kinky back (p. 270).
(6)   Machine damage (p. 270).
(7)   Osteopetrosis (p. 271).
(8)   Rickets (p. 273).
(9)   Tuberculosis (p. 276).

Head

(1)   Blackhead (p. 263).
(2)   Cannibalism (p. 264).
(3)   Erysipelas (p. 265).
(4)   Fowl pox (p. 267).
(5)   Infectious sinusitis (p. 275).

(6) Keratoconjunctivitis (p. 270).
(7) Rickets (p. 273).
(8) Shovel beak (p. 275).
(9) Thrush (p. 276).

Heart

(1) Erysipelas (p. 265).
(2) *Escherichia coli* septicaemia (p. 266).
(3) Gout (p. 268).
(4) Round heart (p. 273).

Joints

(1) Gout (p. 268).
(2) Perosis (p. 272).
(3) Rickets (p. 273).
(4) Synovitis (p. 275).
(5) Twisted leg disease (p. 277).

Kidneys

(1) *Escherichia coli* septicaemia (p. 266).
(2) Myeloid leukosis (p. 262).

Liver

(1)   Avian leukosis complex (p. 262).
(2)   Blackhead (p. 263).
(3)   Coli granuloma (p. 265).
(4)   Erysipelas (p. 265).
(5)   Fatty liver syndrome (p. 266).
(6)   Fowl typhoid (p. 267).
(7)   Gout (p. 268).
(8)   Lymphoid leukosis (p. 262).
(9)   Myeloid leukosis (p. 262).
(10) Pullorum disease (p. 272).
(11) Round heart disease (p. 273).
(12) Ulcerative enteritis (p. 277).
(13) Tuberculosis (p. 276).
(14) Virus hepatitis (p. 277).

Lungs

(1)   Aspergillosis (p. 262).
(2)   *Escherichia coli* septicaemia (p. 266).
(3)   Gapes (p. 268).
(4)   Tuberculosis (p. 276).

Muscle

(1)   Breast blisters (p. 263).
(2)   Bruising (p. 264).
(3)   Cannibalism (p. 264).
(4)   Erysipelas (p. 265).
(5)   Machine damage (p. 270).
(6)   Marek's disease (p. 270).
(7)   Oregon disease (p. 271).
(8)   Putrefaction (p. 273).
(9)   Ruptured gastrocnemius tendons (p. 274).
(10) Tread wounds (p. 276).
(11) Mould (p. 164).

Ovaries, oviduct, etc.

(1)   Egg binding (p. 265).
(2)   Egg peritonitis (p. 265).
(3)   Gumboro disease (p. 269).
(4)   Lymphoid leukosis (p. 262).
(5)   Marek's disease (p. 270).
(6)   Prolapse (p. 272).
(7)   Pullorum disease (p. 272).
(8)   Salpingitis (p. 275).

Skin

(1)   Breast blisters (p. 263).
(2)   Bruising (p. 264).
(3)   Bumble foot (p. 264).
(4)   Cannibalism (p. 264).
(5)   Erysipelas (p. 265).
(6)   Fowl pox (p. 267).
(7)   Freezer burn (p. 268).
(8)   Gangrenous dermatitis (p. 268).
(9)   Hernia (p. 269).
(10) Machine damage (p. 270).

(11)   Marek's disease (p. 270).
(12)   Mould (p. 164).
(13)   Plantar necrosis (p. 272).
(14)   Putrefaction (p. 273).
(15)   Red mite (p. 273).
(16)   Scaly leg (p. 275).
(17)   Tissue mites (p. 276).
(18)   Xanthomatosis (p. 277).

Spleen

(1)   Avian leukosis complex (p. 262).
(2)   Erysipelas (p. 265)
(3)   Tuberculosis (p. 276).

Stomach and intestines

(1)   Blackhead (p. 263).
(2)   Coccidiosis (p. 264).
(3)   Fowl typhoid (p. 267).
(4)   Hexamitiasis (p. 267).
(5)   Newcastle disease (p. 266).
(6)   Prolapse (p. 272).
(7)   Pullorum disease (p. 272).
(8)   Pustular typhylitis (p. 272).
(9)   Roundworms (p. 274).
(10)   Thrush (p. 276).
(11)   Tuberculosis (p. 276).
(12)   Ulcerative enteritis (p. 277).

Appendix 1
Legislation

The Food Safety Act 1990
The Animal Health Act 1981
The Fresh Meat (Hygiene and Inspection) Regulations 1995, amended by
  The Fresh Meat (Hygiene and Inspection) (Amendment) Regulations 1995
  The Fresh Meat (Hygiene and Inspection) (Amendment) Regulations 1996
The Welfare of Animals (Slaughter or Killing) Regulations 1995
The Animal By-Products (Identification) Regulations 1995
The Specified Bovine Material (No. 3) Order 1996
The Bovine Offal (Prohibition) Regulations 1989, amended by
  The Bovine Offal (Prohibition) (Amendment) Regulations 1992
  The Bovine Offal (Prohibition) (Amendment) Regulations 1994
  The Bovine Offal (Prohibition) (Amendment) Regulations 1995
The Bovine Spongiform Encephalopathy Order 1996, amended by
  The Bovine Spongiform Encephalopathy (Amendment) Order 1996
The Fresh Meat (Beef Control) (No 2) Regulations 1996, amended by
  The Fresh Meat (Beef Control) (No 2) (Amendment) Regulations 1996
The Heads of Sheep and Goats Order 1996
The Cattle Passports Order 1996
The Meat Products (Hygiene) Regulations 1994
The Poultry Meat, Farmed Game Bird Meat and Rabbit Meat (Hygiene and Inspection) Regulations 1995
The Wild Game Meat (Hygiene and Inspection) Regulations 1995
The Minced Meat and Meat Preparations (Hygiene) Regulations 1995
The Food Safety (General Food Hygiene) Regulations 1995
The Food Safety (Temperature Control) Regulations 1995

Appendix 2
Colloquial Terms

Australian crop or pony	Forequarter beef less brisket and shin
Back fat	Subcutaneous fat from back of pig
Baron of beef	Twin sirloins undivided
Bible	Omasum
Blade bone	Scapula
Bobby calf	Young calf
Book	Omasum
Brocks	Edible offals
Buff	Lungs
Bung or bung gut	Caecum
Calf bed	Uterus
Calf vell	Calf abomasum
Camel hair	Ligamentum nuchae
Catch bag	Uterus
Caul fat	Omentum (kell)
Closed side	Right side of beef (**NB** kidney fixed in loin)
Clynes	Lymph nodes
Cod fat	Scrotal fat
Crow or crown fat	Mesenteric fat of pig (mudgeon)
Crup fat	Omental fat
Dough or dugg	Udder fat of maiden females
Dredlock	Unthrifty pig
Farthing	Omasum
Fell	To slaughter
FK	Fresh killed
Gambrel	Small pork pig, or length of iron on which it hangs
Geeshead	Genital organs or male urinary organs
Glove fat	Peritoneal fat of pig (leaf)
Golden slippers	Untrodden feet of fetus (bovine)
Gowel	Symphysis pubis
Greaves	Residue from rendering of pork fat – scratchings
Gullet	Oesophagus (weasand or wasund)

Gut bread	Pancreas
Hanging side	Describes left side with floating kidney
HK	Home killed
H-bone	Tuber coxae
Harple bone	Atlas, 1st cervical vertebra
Heart bread	Thymus
Hodge	Cooked-pig's stomach
Honeycomb	Reticulum
Kell	Omentum (caul)
Kernels	Lymph nodes
Lamb's fry	Lamb's testicles
Leaf	Peritoneal fat – pig (glove fat)
Leaf seam	Peritoneal fat – pig (glove fat)
Lites	Lungs
Lying side	Right side with fixed kidney
Manyplies	Omasum
Mate	Sheep and pig mesentery
Maw	Uncooked pig's stomach
Melt	Speen (milt or smelt)
Milt	Spleen
Mudgeon	Mesenteric fat of pig – crow or crown fat
Open side	Left side of beef – raison side
Oxter	Where the underside of the leg and flank meet
Pare	Trim off fat
Paunch	Ruminant stomachs
Pig's fry	Larynx, trachea, lungs, oesophagus, heart and liver, spleen and omentum
Pig's pluck	Larynx, trachea, lungs, oesophagus, heart and liver, spleen and omentum
Pig's frytop	Fry less liver
Pin bone	Tuber ischii
Pluck, sheep or calf	Trachea, lungs, heart and liver
Psalterium	Omasum
Raice	Sheep or calf pluck
Raison side	Open side of beef
Raps	Small intestines – ropes or runners
Reed	Abomasum
Rig	Male pig with one undescended testicle
Rind	Skin of pig
Roll	Oesophagus
Ropes	Small intestines – runners
Runners	Small intestines – ropes
Runt	Small unthrifty pig
Scratchings	Residue from rendering pork fat–greaves

Skins	Intestines
Skirt	Diaphragm
Slink	Fetal calf
Smelt	Spleen
Stag	Male bovine or male pig castrated late
Stick	To bleed
TK	Town killed
Target	Sheep forequarter less shoulder
Thrapple	Larynx and trachea
Throat bread	Thymus
Vell	Calf abomasum
Wasund	Oesophagus – gullet or weasand
Weasand	Oesophagus – gullet or wasund
Web	Ox mesentery
Willdew	Pig with mixture of male and female genital organs, i.e. hermaphrodite

Bibliography

1. *The Lancet* Vol. 347, 6 April 1996.
2. Spongiform Encephalopathy Advisory Committee advice on sheep. MAAF Press Release 271/96.
3. Spongiform Encephalopathy Advisory Committee statement on the new strain of CJD, 20 March 1996.
4. Spongiform Encephalopathy Advisory Committee statement on BSE, 24 March 1996.
5. Spongiform Encephalopathy Advisory Committee statement on maternal transmission, 1 August 1996.
6. Spongiform Encephalopathy Advisory Committee statement on BSE and the environment, 7 June 1996.
7. Pearson, A.D. & Healing, T.D. The surveillance and control of *Campylobacter* infection. *Communicable Disease Report* **2**, Review Number 12, 6 November 1992.
8. PHLS Vero cytotoxin-producing *Escherichia coli* O157 Factsheet, 7 January 1997.

Index

ACTH, 75
abdomen, 15
abnormal colour, 105
  conditions, 99
  odours, 102
  pigmentations, 105
abomasal and intestinal
  ulceration, 190
abomasum, 52
abortion
  contagious (bovine
    brucellosis), 123
  due to chlamydia, 125
  due to listeria, 129
  due to sarcocysts, 157
  due to toxoplasma, 156
abscess, 104
  poultry, 261
Acaridae (mites), 162
acetonaemia (ketosis), 103
acetone, 103
  Rothera's test for, 103
  smell of, 103
Achromobacter, 203
actinobacillosis, 115
Actinobacillus lignieresi,
  115
Actinomyces
  bovis, 116
  israeli, 116
  suis, 116
actinomycosis, 116
Addison's disease, 77
adenoma, 192
adenosine diphosphate
  (ADP), 1
adenosine triphosphate
  (ATP), 1, 85
adipokinen, 75
adipose tissue, 3
adrenal glands, 77
adrenaline, 77
aflatoxicosis, 261

afterfeather, 241
age estimation, 94
  calves, 95
  cattle, 94
  deer, 96
  horse, 96
  pig, 95
  poultry, 237
  sheep, 95
air chamber, 255
  sacs, 251
  sacculitis, 261
aldosterone, 77
alimentary canal, 49
  accessory organs, 55
ambiens muscle, 246
amylase, 49
anaemia, 167
Anaplocephala, 147
anasarca, 100
anatomy of fowl, 241
angioma, 176
ankylosing spondylitis, 170
ante-mortem inspection, 86
anterior chamber, 73
anthracosis, 105
anthrax, 116
apteria, 241
aqueous humour, 73
arachnoid, 71
areolar tissue, 3
arteries, 26
arthritis, 173
Arthropoda, 140, 158
arytenoid cartilage, 43
Ascaridia
  dissimilis, 274
  galli, 274
Ascaris
  lumbricoides, 141
  suum, 141
ascites, 105, 261
aspergillosis, 262

Aspergillus
  flavis, 165
  fumigatus, 166, 262
atrophic rhinitis, 171
  in rabbit, 231
atrophy, 194
  brown, 105
auditory ossicles, 74
auricle, 25, 74
avian leukosis complex, 262
  tuberculosis, 135, 276
azoturia, 118

Babesia divergens, 158
babesiasis, 158
bacillary necrosis, 177
  white diarrhoea (BWD),
    263
Bacillus anthracis, 116
Bacillus mallei, 127
back bleeding, 84, 181
bacon
  carcass preparation, 212
  curing, 210, 215
  cuts, 214
  dry curing, 218
  glazy, 106
  grading, 211
  smoking, 217
  Wiltshire, 212
bacteraemia, 111
bacteria, 110
  in ruminant digestion, 49
  pathogenic, 110
  saprophytic, 112
bacterial necrosis, 177
Bacteroides necrophorus,
  123, 177, 187
badgers, tuberculosis in,
  136
barbs, 241
barbules, 241
beak necrosis, 275

bicuspid valve, 25
big liver disease, 262
bile, 49
bile staining, 115
bilirubin, 49
biliverdin, 49
bites
    in muntjac bucks, 188
    in pigs, 186, 187
black pudding, 220
black spot, 165
blackhead, 263
blackleg, 118
blackquarter, 118
bladder, 62
blast freezing, 205
bleeding, 83
    imperfect, 100
    insufficiency, 100
    of poultry, 257
blood, 24
    affections of, 167
    amount at slaughter, 83
    circulation, 26
        fetal, 29
    clotting, 24
    splashing, 83, 180
    from anthrax infected
        carcasses, 117
blood vessels, 26
blow flies, 161
blown-canned goods, 209
blue green mould, 165
bluebottles, 161
body cavities, 14
body temperatures, 87
boiling test, 103, 167
bone, 4
    affections of, 169
    differential features,
        16–20
    in leaf fat of pigs, 112
    of skeletal system, 11
    taint, 103
    tissue, 4
Bordatella bronchiseptica,
    233
botriomycosis, 118
botulism, 227
bovine spongiform
    encephalopathy
    (BSE),118

bovine virus diarrhoea, 123
bow legged deformity, 272
bowel oedema, 190
brain, 71
    cysts in, 150
    structure, 71
brawn, 222
breast blisters, 263
brine, 216
    staining, 105
brown atrophy, 105
brown fat, 4
Brucella
    abortus, 123
    melitensis, 123
    suis, 123
brucellosis, 123
bruising, 100
    of poultry, 264
bulbo-urethral glands, 64
bumble foot, 264
bursa of Fabricius, 249
    lesions in, 260, 270
butchers' joints, 196–201
button ulcers, 134

caecal tonsils, 248
calamus, 241
calcification, presternal,
    194
calf, age of, 95
    diptheria, 123
    immaturity of, 95
Calliphora erythrocephala,
    161
    vomitora, 161
Camphylobacter jejuni, 225
cancer, 192
Candida albicans, 276
canicola fever, 128
cannibalism, 264
canning, 206
    spoilage, 208
Capillaria, 234
capillaries, 26
capine arthritis
        encephalitis, 124
captive bolt pistols, 82
carbon dioxide, 203
    anaesthesia, 83
carcasses
    definition, 88

electrical stimulation, 87
fevered, 101
hot boning of, 88
immature, 102
joints, 196–201
lymph nodes, 33–41
sex characteristics and
    differentiation of, 89
carcinoma, 192
carotene, 3, 105, 107
cartilage, 4
    of the larynx, 43
caseation, 112
caseous lymphadenitis, 124
castor, bean tick, 164
cat, bone compared with
    rabbit, 16
cattle
    affections of
        blood, 167
        bones, 169
        head and tongue, 170
        heart, 172
        joints, 173
        kidney, 174
        liver, 176
        lungs and pleura, 179
        lymph nodes, 182
        mammary glands, 183
        muscles, 184
        skin, 187
        spleen, 188
        stomach and intestines,
            189
        udder, 183
        uterus, 191
    age estimation of, 94
    bones compared with
        horse, 16
    endocrine glands, 75
    fat, characteristics of, 3
    head, 43
    heart, 27
    horns, 94
    intestine length, 54
    kidneys, 62
    larynx, 43
    liver, 55
    lymph nodes, 35–9
    lymphatic system, 32
    mouth and tongue, 50
    pancreas, 58

pelvis, 14
physiological
    characteristics, 87
sex, characteristics of
    carcass, 89
skeleton, 13
slaughter of, 83
spleen, 59
stomachs, 52
teeth, 94
testicles, 65
tonsils, 52
trachea and lungs, 44
uterus, 68
vertebrae, 12
catty odour, 102
cavernous haemangioma,
    176
cells, 1
Cepheneymia, 160
central nervous system,
    71–2
cerebellum, 72
cerebrum, 72
cestodes, 146
    of poultry, 276
chalaza, 255
cheesy odour, 103
chickens, categories of,
    237–8
chilling of meat, 203
    of pultry, 258
Chalymidia psittaci, 125
chitterlings, 221
chondroma, 192
chorioid, 73
chorionic gonadotrophine,
    77
chorioptes, 164
chorioptic mange, 164
chromosomes, 1
chronic venous congestion,
    188
chyle, 32
ciliary muscle, 73
circulation, blood, 26
    fetal, 29
circulatory system, 24–30
cirrhosis, 177
    hypertrophic, 178
Cladosporium herbarum
    165, 271

cloaca, 240
cloacal bursa, 249
close seasons, deer, 7
Clostridium
    botulinum, 227
    chauvoei, 118
    perfringens, 103, 202, 268
    putrefaciens, 103
    tetani, 135
clotting, blood, 24
Cnemidocoptes mutans, 275
coccidia and coccidiosis,
    156
    of poultry, 264
    of rabbits, 231
Coenurus
    cerebralis, 150
    serialis, 151, 231
cold shortening, 204
coli granuloma, 265
colloquial terms, 283
colour, abnormal, 105
commensals, 109
conjunctiva, 73
connective tissues, 3
    parasitic nematodes of,
    145
contagious abortion, 123
contagious catarrh, 232, 233
contagious pustular
    dermatitis, 130
contamination of lungs, 179
    of trachea, 179
cooked products, 222
coprodeum, 248
cornea, 73
corned beef, 206
coronary furrow, 25
corticortisone, 77
corticotrophin, 75
Corynebacterium
    equi, 183
    ovis, 124
    pyogenes, 183
cotyledons, 68
cow pox, 184
Coxiella burnetti, 110
cranial cavity, 14
crest, 91
cretinism, 76
cricoid cartilage, 43
crop, 246

Culicoides pungens, 145
curled toe
    paralysis, 265
    syndrome, 265
Cyclops strenuus, 153
cysterni chyli, 32
Cysticercus
    bovis, 152
    cellulosae, 152
    echinococcus, 149
    ovis, 150
    pisiformis, 151, 232
    tenuicollis, 149
cysts
    coenurus, 150
    congenital, 174
    echinococcus, 149
    hydronephrosis, 174
    sarcocysts, 157
    trichinella spiralis, 143
cytoplasm, 1

Damalinia ovis, 162
dark cutting beef, 106
dark firm and dry pork
    (DFD), 106
Davinia proglottina, 276
deer and venison, 6
    actinomycosis, 116
    age of, 96
    anthrax, 116
    Aspergillus fumigatus,
    166
    bleeding of, 84
    body temperature, 87
    bones, 16
    Cephenemyia auribrabus,
    158, 160
        stimulator, 158, 160
    close seasons, 7
    coccidia, 156
    Cysticercus tenuicollis,
    149
    dentition, 96
    Dictyocaulus viviparus,
    144
    echinococcus cysts, 148
    Elaphostrongylus cervi,
    145
    Fasciola hepatica, 153
    foot and mouth disease,
    125

gestation, 7
gralloch, 6
haemonchus, 141
Haemophysalis punctata, 164
head, affections of, 171
heart
    differential features, 29
Hydrotoea irritans, 161
Hypoderma diana, 158
hydronephrosis, 174
intestines, affections of, 190
    parasites of, 142
Ixodes ricinus, 158
Johne's disease, 127
joints of, 200
ked, 160
kidneys, affections of, 176
    differential features, 64
leptospirosis, 128
listeriosis, 129
liver, affections of, 178
    differential features, 58
Lipoptema cervi, 160
lung worms, 144
lungs, affections of, 181
    differentiation of, 46
lymph nodes, 39
    affections of, 183
malignant fever, 130
Muellarius capillaris, 145
muscle, affections of, 185
mycotic pneumonia, 166
nasal flies, 158, 160
Nematodirus battus, 142
    follicollis, 142
Ostertagia, 141
pleura, affections of, 181
Protostrongylus rufescens, 145
pulse, 87
reindeer, 8
respiratory rate, 87
Sarcocystis wapiti, 157
sexual odour, 102
shooting of, 6
skin, affections of, 188
slaughter of, 6
species, 7
spleen, affections of, 189

    differential features, 60
stomachs, affections of, 190
    terms, 7
    testicles, differential features, 67
ticks, 164
tongue, affections of, 171
    differential features, 51
trichostrongyles, 141
tuberculosis, 138
uterus, differential features of, 69
winter death syndrome, 100
Yersinia psudotuberculosis, 139
yersiniosis, 139
defeathering, 257
degenerative myopathy, 271
demodectic mange, 164
Demodex, 164
dental pad, 49
deoxyribonucleic acid (DNA), 1
Dermacentor reticulatus, 164
Dermanyssus gallinae, 273
Dermestes lardarius, 161
diabetes, 76
diamonds, 133
diaphragm, 14
diaphragmatic hernia, 189
Diaptomus gracilis, 153
diarrhoea
    and Johne's disease, 127
    and salmonellosis, 132
Diacrocelium dendriticum, 155
Dictyocaulus arnfieldi, 144
    filaria, 144
    viviperus, 144
digestive system, 48–61
    of fowl, 246
dipeptidase, 49
Diphyllobhothrium latum, 153
disease, 109
    immunity, 113
    of poultry, 261

of rabbits, 231
    parasitic, 140
dislocation, 173
dogs, tapeworms of, 148
double muscles, 193
drainage areas, 31
drenching gun injuries, 170
dressing
    of poultry, 258
drip, 204
driving sickness, 131
dropsy, 101, 261
ductless glands, 75
ductus arteriosus, 30
ductus deferens, 64
ductus venosus, 30
duodenum, 54
dura mater, 71

ear, 73
    damage to, 171
    haematoma of, 171
    of fowl, 252
    structure, 73
Echinococcus granulosus, 148
    cysts, 148
egg, anatomy of, 254
    binding, 265
    peritonitis, 265
Eimeria, 156, 231
Elaphostrongylus cervi, 145
elastic tissue, 3
electrical stimulation, 87
electrical stunning, 82
emaciation, 100, 265
emergency slaughter, 85
emphysema, 179
    interlobular, 179
    interestitial, 179
    intestinal, 190
    mesenteric, 190
endocarditis, 172
    verrucose, 133
endocrine system, 75, 251
endothelium, 26
enteritis, 124, 133
enzootic abortion of ewes, 125
enzootic bovine leukosis, 125
enzootic pneumonia, 125

enzymes, digestive, 48
eosinophilic myositis, 106
epicarditis, 173
epicardium, 25
epididymis, 65
epiglottic cartilage, 43
epithelium, 2
erepsin, 49
epithelial tissues, 2
erysipelas
    of fowl, 265
    swine, 133
erysipeloid, 133
erysipelothrix
    insidiosa, 133, 265
    rhusiopathiae, 133, 265,
        275
erythema, transit, 186
erythoid leukosis, 253
erythroblastosis, 263
erythrocytes, 24
Escherichia coli, 249
Escherichia coli
    septicaemia, 266
Eustachian tube, 74
evisceration of poultry, 257
ewe, differentiation from
    goat, 92
exhaustion, 114
exophthalmus, 76
expiration, 42
exsanguination, 83
external auditory meatus,
    73
eye, 72
    structure, 72

faecal contamination, 104
fallopian tubes, 67
farcy, 127
Fasciola hepatica, 153
fasciolaisis, 153
fat, 3
    back fat measurement,
        211
    bone plates in, 112
    brown, 4
    characteristics of, 3
    lard, 221
    pigmentation, 105, 107,
        109, 234
fat necrosis, 194, 266

fatty change, 176
fatty liver syndrome, 266
feathers, 241
febrile disease, and pH
    measurement, 114
fetal
    circulation, 29
    flesh, 101
fevered flesh, 101
fibrin, 25
fibroma, 192
fibroplastic nephritis, 175
fibrous tissue, 4
flipper, 209
flukes, 153
fluky liver, 155
fly blown, 161
fly strike, 161
food poisoning, 225
foot and mouth disease, 125
foramen orale, 30
Formica fusta, 155
foul of foot, 187
fowl
    anatomy of, 241–55
    bones compared with
        rabbit, 18
    diseases, 261–77
    paralysis, 266, 270
    pest, 266
    plague, 267
    pox, 267
    skeleton, 242
    typhoid, 267
fractures, 169
freezer burn, 106, 206, 268
fungi, 110
    parasitic, 166

gad flies, 158
gadding, 158
Galumna, 146
gall bladder, 55
gammon, 215
gangrene, 112
gangrenous dermatitis, 268
gapes, 268
gastric juice, 48
gastrocnemius tendons,
    ruptured, 274
gastroenteritis, 232
    parasitic, 232

Gastrophilus intestinalis,
    160
genital organs, 64–70
    of fowl, 252–5
gestation periods, 87
gid, 150
gizzard, 246
glanders, 127
glands
    bulbo-urethral, 64
    ductless, 75
    mammary, 67
    of endocrine system, 75–8
    of eye, 72
    prostate, 64
Glässer's disease, 127
glazy bacon, 106
glucagon, 76
goats
    bones compared with
        sheep, 16
    carcass compared with
        sheep, 92
    characteristics of fat, 3
    mouth and tongue, 49, 50
    physiological
        characteristics, 87
    skin odours, 102
    spleen, 59
goitre, 76
golden slippers, 101
golgi bodies, 1
gout, fowl, 268
gralloch, 6
'grapes', 138
Graphidium strigosum, 232
gristle, 4
gullet, 49
Gumboro disease, 269

haemal lymph node, 33
haemangioma, cavernous,
    176
Haemaphysalis punctata,
    164
haematoma, 101
Haematopinus, 162
haemoglobinaemia, 168
Haemonchus contortus,
    141
Haemophilus suis, 127
haemosporidia, 158

halál, 85
ham
  canned, 208
  cooked, 222
  York, 218
ham beetle, 161
head and tongue, affections
  of, 170–71
heart, 25, 27–9
  affections of, 172–3
heart bread, 77
heat preseration, 206
heparin, 24
hepatitis, viral, of ducks, 277
hernia, 269
Heterakis gallinarum, 263
hexamitiasis, 269
Histomonas meleagridis,
  263
histomoniasis, 269
Hjärre's disease, 265
hoose, 144
hormones, 75
horns, ageing by, 94
horse bot fly, 158, 160
horses
  age estimation, 96
  bones compared with ox,
    16
  fat characteristics, 3
  heart, 28
  intestine length, 54
  kidney, 63
  liver, 57
  lungs, 46
  lymph nodes, 41
  mouth and tongue, 51
  physiological
    characteristics, 87
  spleen, 60
  stomach, 54
  teeth, 96
  testicles, 66
  tonsils, 52
  trachea and lungs, 46
  uterus, 69
  vertebral formula, 12
hot deboning, 88
husk, 144
hyaline cartilage, 4
hydatid cyst, 148
  disease, 148

sand, 149
hydraemia, 168
hydrochloric acid, 48
hydrocortisone, 77
hydrogen ion
  concentration, 113
hydronephrosis, 174
hydropericardium, 100
Hydrotaea irritans, 161
hydrothorax, 100
Hyostrongulus rubidus, 142
hypernephroma, 175
hypertrophic cirrhosis, 178
hypertrophy, 193
hyphae, 110
hypocalcaemia, 168
Hypoderma
  aeratum, 158
  bovis, 158
  diana, 158
  lineatum, 158
hypomagnesaemia, 168
hypothyroidism, 76

icterus, 107
  of fowl, 269
immaturity, 102
immunity, 113
imperfect bleeding, 100
incus, 73
infandibulum, 253
infarcts, 175
infection, 110
infectious bronchitis, 269
infectious enterohepatitis,
  263
infectious
  keratoconjunctivitis,
  128
infectious sinusitis, 269
infectious synovitis, 275
inflammation, 104
injection coloration, 107
inspiration, 42
insufficiency of bleeding,
  100
insulin, 76
interarytenoid cartilage, 45
interlobular emphysema,
  179
interestitial emphysema,
  179

interestitial myositis, 184
intervertebral discs, 12
intestinal emphysema, 190
intestinal juice, 49
intestines, 54
  affections of, 189–190
  of fowl, 246
  secretions, 48
  structure and lengths, 54
intrascope, 211
invertase, 49
iodine, in diet, 76
iris, 72
islets of Langerhans, 76
isthmus, 253
Ixodes ricinus, 158

Jaagsiekte, 131
jaundice, 107
  of fowl, 269
  test for, 105
jaws, 11
jelly, 223
Jewish slaughter, 84
Johne's disease, 127
joint ill, 173, 177
joints, 20
  affections of, 173–4
  beef, 197, 198
  butchers', 196
  lamb, 199
  pork, 201
  venison, 200
judgement, 97

keds, 160
keel, 245
keratitis, 128
keratoconjunctivitis, 128,
  270
ketosis, 103
kidney worm, 146
kidneys, 62
  affections of, 174–6
  of fowl, 252
kinky back, 270
knock-kneed deformity,
  272
kosher, 84

lacrimal gland, 72
lactase, 49

lacteals, 32
lairage, 86
lamb and mutton joints, 199
Laminosioptes cysticola, 276
lard, 221
larval infection of meat, 161
larynx, 42
leaf, 221
leatherhead, 265
legislation, 282
lens, 72
leptospirosis, 128
leucocytes, 24
leukaemia, 168
leukosis, avian, 261
lice, 162
licked back, 159
ligaments, 22
    abdominal 61
    bone, 4, 11
ligamentum nuchae, 3, 22, 43
lime burning, 156
line slaughter, 87
Linguatula serrata, 155, 161
Linognathus, 162
    ovis, 162
lipase, 48, 49
lipofuchsinosis, 105
lipoma, 192
lipomatosis of muscle, 184
Liponyssius caponis, 162
Lipoptema cervi, 160
Listeria monocytogenes, 129, 226
listeriosis, 129, 226
liver, 55–8
    abscess, 177
    affections of, 176–9
    fluke, 153
    focal necrosis of, 177
    sawdust, 177
lockjaw, 135
long legged poultry, 259
Lucilia sericata, 160
lumpy jaw, 116
lung oedema, 270
lung worms, 144
lujngs, 43–7
    affections of, 179–81
    contamination, 180

fetal, 44
    in poultry, 250
luteinising hormone, 75
Lymnea truncatula, 154
lymph, 31–41
    nodes, 33
    affections of, 182–3
lymphadenitis, 129
lymphatic system, 31–41
    tissue, 3
lymphoid leucosis, 262
lymphoid tissue, 3
lymphosarcoma, 192
lysosomes, 2

machine damage, 104
    fowl, 270
    pig, 104
Maedi-Visna, 129
maggots, 161
magnum, 253
malignant aptha, 130
malignant catarrhal fever, 130
malignat pustule, 116
malignant tumours, 192
malleus, 73
Malphighian corpuscles, 59
Malta fever, 123
maltase, 49
mammary glands, 67
    affections of, 183–4
mange, 162
marble bone, 271
marble spleen disease, 270
marbling, 3
Marek's disease, 270
marrow, 5
'master' gland, 75
mastitis, 183
meat
    canning of, 206
    chilling of, 203
    definition of, 88
    extract, 208
    preservation, 202, 206
    products, 202
    spoilage of, 202, 208, 225
    thawing of, 205
Mecanthus stramineus, 162
mechanical stunning, 81

medulla oblongata, 71
melanocyte, 75
melanosis, 107
melatonin, 78
Melophagus ovinus, 160
meninges, 71
mesenteric emphysema, 190
mesentery, 61
mesityl oxide, 102
mesophiles, 202
metaplasia, 112
metastasis, 193
Metastrongylus, 145
    apri, 145
    pudendotectus, 145
    salmi, 145
metritis, 196
micro-organism, 109
microvilli, 2
Miescher's tubes, 157
migratory flukes, 155
miliary tuberculosis, 138
'milk spot', 141
milk fever, 168
mites, 162
mitochondria, 1
Moniezia benedini, 147
    expanza, 146
moniliasis, 276
Morexella bovis, 128
moulds, 164, 202, 271
mouth, 49
    affections of, 170–71
    of fowl, 246
mucoid enteritis, 232
mucosal disease, 130
Muellerius capillaris, 145
Multiceps
    multiceps, 150
    serialis, 151
mummified fetus, 191
muscle, 23
muscle, 23
    affections of, 184–5
    double, 193
    fat marbling in, 3
    lipomatosis, 184
    of poultry, 245
muscular fibrosis, 184
    hypertrophy, 193
    system, 23

Muslim slaughter, 85
mycelium, 110
Mycobacterium
  avium, 136
  bovis, 136
  intracellularae, 136
  johnei, 127
  tuberculosis, 136
Mycoplasma
  conjunctivae, 128
  gallisepticum, 261
  hypopneumoniae, 125
  synoviae, 261, 275
myeloid leukosis, 262
myocarditis, 173
myxoedema, 76
myxomatosis, 232

necrobacillosis, 177
necrosis, 112
  of beaks, 275
  of fat, 169, 266
  of pigs' tails, 187
  plantar, 272
necrotic enteritis, 131
nematodes, 140
  of poultry, 274
nematodirus, 142
nephritis, fibroplastic, 175
nephritis, pyelo, 175
nephritis, rabbits, 232
nervous system, 71, 251
New York Dressed poultry
  (NYD), 259
Newcastle disease, 271
nictitating membrane, 252
nitrate poisoning, 108
nitrite poisoning, 108
nitroso-haemoglobin, 216
nodular necrosis, 185
noradrenaline, 77
nostril, fly, sheep, 160
not yet dressed poultry, 259
nucleolus, 1
nucleoplasm, 1
nucleus, 1

ochronosis, 108
odours, abnormal, 102
oedema, 100
Oesophagostomum
  columbianum, 142

  dentatum, 142
  radiatum, 142
oesophagus, 49
oestradiol, 77
oestrogens, 77
oestrone, 77
Oestrus ovis, 160
offal, definition of, 80
oil gland, 241
olein, 3
omasum, 52
omentum, 61
Onchocerca gibsoni, 145
  guttorosa, 146
onchocerciasis, 145
Oregon disease, 271
orf, 130
os coxae, 12
ossa cordis, 27, 28
ossifying spondylitis, 170
oesteohaemato-
  chromatocis, 108, 169
osteoma, 192
osteomalacia, 169
osteomyelitis, 116
oesteopetrosis, 271
Ostertagia ostertagi, 141
ovaries, 77
  of fowl, 253
oversticking, 94, 181
oviduct, 253

pH, 113
Paget's disease, 271
palate, 49
pale soft exudate (PSE),
  108
palmitin, 3
pancreas, 52, 76
pancreatic juice, 49, 76
panniculus adiposus, 3
papilloma, 192
Paramphistomum cervi,
  153, 156
paramyxovirus, 271
Parascaris equorum, 141
parasites, 140
parasitic diseases, 140
  arthropoda, 158
  fungi, 166
  protozoa, 156
  worms, 141

parasitic gastroenteritis,
  141
  of rabbits, 232
parathormone, 76
parathyroid glands, 76
paratuberculosis, 127
pathology, 97
Passalurus ambiguus, 232
Pasteurella multocida, 232
pastry, 223
patagium, 241
pelvic bones, 12
pelvis, 13, 15
  of fowl, 244
Penicillium, 166
penis, 64
pentastomes, 161
pepsin, 48
peptic ulcers, 189
periarteritis nodosa, 172
pericardial fluid, 25
pericarditis, traumatic, 173
pericardium, 25
periosteum, 4
peritoneum, 61
peritonitis, 188
perosis, 272
petechial haemorrhages,
  174, 175
pharynx, 49
phosphorescence, 108
physiological data, 87
pia mater, 71
pies, 223
pig paratyphoid, 131
pigmentation, abnormal,
  105
pigs
  affections of
    bones, 169
    head and tongue, 171
    heart, 173
    joints, 174
    kidney, 175
    liver, 178
    lungs, 180
    lymph nodes, 182
    muscles, 185
    skin, 186
    spleen, 189
    stomach and intestines,
      190

udder, 184
uterus, 191
age estimation, 95
fat characteristics, 3
heart, 28
intestine length, 54
kidney, 63
liver, 56
lungs, 45
lymph nodes, 40
machine damage to, 104
odour from boars, 102
pancreas, 58
physiological
    characteristics, 87
sex characteristics of
    carcasses, 92–4
slaughter, 84
spleen, 60
stomach, 53
teeth, 95
testicles, 65
thyroid gland, 76
tongue, 50
tonsils, 52
trachea and lungs, 45
uterus, 69
vertebral formula, 12
pimply gut, 142
pineal gland, 78
pink eye, 128
pipy liver, 155
pithing, 82
pituitary gland, 75
pityriasis rosea, 186
placenta, 77
plantar necrosis, 272
plasma, 24
platelets, 24
plerocercoid, 153
pleura, 47
    affections of, 179–81
pleural fluid, 47
pleurisy, 179
pneumonia, 179, 180
    enzootic, 180
    in rabbits, 233
    virus, 125
polony, 220
polyarteritis, 172
polyathritis, 173
polyphosphate, 258

pons, 72
poorness, 100
pork
    brawn, 222
    joints, 201
    pies, 223
    stress syndrome, 108
posterior chamber, 73
post-mortem inspection, 86,
    259
poultry
    affections of specific
        parts, 278–81
    anatomy, 241–5
    bleeding of, 251
    chilling of, 258
    defeathering, 257
    definitions, 237–40
    diseases of, 261–77
    dressing of, 258
    evisceration, 257
    freezing, 259
    fresh chilled, 259
    inspection, 259
    legislation, 256
    scalding, 257
    skeleton, 242
    slaughter, 256
    stunning, 256
preening, 241
pregnancy table, 87
    toxaemia, 191
preservation of meat, 203
    cold, 203
    heat, 206
presternal calcification, 194
primary lesion, 111
procercoid, 153
proctodeum, 249
progesterone, 77
prolactin, 75
prolapse, 272
prostate, 64
prothrombin, 24
protoplasm, 1
Protostrongylus rufescens,
    145
protozoa, 110, 140
proventriculus, 246
Przhevalskiana silenus, 158
Pseudomonas
    phosphoescence, 108

Psoroptes, 163
    communis ovis, 163
psoroptic mange, 163
psychrophiles, 202
pterylae, 241
ptyalin, 48
pullorum disease, 272
pulmonary adenomatosis,
    131
pulse rates, 87
pustular typhiltis, 272
putrefaction, 272
putty brisket, 194
pyaemia, 111
pyaemic abscesses, 111
pyelonephritis, 175
pygostyle, 19, 243
pyometra, 191

'Q' (query) fever, 131
quadrigemina, 72
quail disease, 277
quill, 242

rabbits
    bones compared with cat
        and fowl, 16
    diseases of, 231–3
    slaughter, 231
    syphilis, 223
rabies, 132
rachis, 241
Raillietina echinobothrida,
    276
    tetragona, 276
Rainey's corpuscles, 157
red mite, 273
redwater, 158
regenerative hyperplasia,
    178
reindeer, 8
rennet, 60
rennin, 48
respiration rates, 87
respiratory system, 43
    of fowl, 250
reticular tissue, 3
reticulitis, traumatic, 189
reticulum, 52
retina, 73
rheumatism, 173
ribonucleic acid (RNA), 1

ribosomes, 1
ribs, 12
rickets, 273
rickettsiae, 110
rigor mortis, 3, 85
Rimmington and Fowrie
    test, 105
ringworm, 166
ritual slaughter, 84
    of poultry, 256
Roekl's granuloma, 185
Rothera's test, 103
round heart disease, 273
roundworms, 140
    of poultry, 274
    of rabbits, 232
rumen, 52
rupture, fowl, 269
ruptured gastrocnemius
    tendons, 274

sacrum, 12
saliva, 48
salivary glands, 48
salmonella food poisoning,
    226
salmonella of poultry, 274
Salmonella cholerae suis,
    132
    dublin, 132
    enteritidis, 132, 274
    gallinarum, 274
    pullorum, 274
    typhimurium, 132, 274
salmonellosis, 132
salpingitis, 275
sapraemia, 112
saprophytic bacteria, 123
Sarcocystis
    bertrami, 157
    capricornis, 157
    cruzi, 157
    equicanis, 157
    fusiformis, 157
    gigantea, 157
    hiricanis, 157
    hominis, 157
    miescheriana, 157
    mouléi, 157
    ovicanis, 157
    porcifilis, 157
    suihominis, 157

tenella, 157
wapiti, 157
sarcocysts, 157
sarcolemma, 23
sarcoma, 192
sarcoptes scabei, 162
sarcoptic mange, 162
sausage, 218
    casings, 219
    manufacture of, 218
    slime on, 203
sawdust liver, 177
scalding, 257
scaly leg, 275
sclera, 73
scrapie, 133
searching, 84
secretin, 77
seedy belly, 107
semicircular canals, 74
seminal vesicles, 64
septic mastitis, 183
septicaemia, 111
septum, 25
serratia, 202
serum, 24
sex characteristics, 89
sexual odour, 102
shechita, 84
sheep
    affections of
        bones, 169
        head and tongue, 170
        heart, 172
        joints, 174
        kidney, 175
        liver, 177
        lungs, 180
        lymph nodes, 182
        mammary glands, 184
        muscle, 185
        skin, 187
        spleen, 188
        stomach and intestines,
            190
        udder, 184
        uterus, 191
    age estimation, 95
    bones compared with
        goat, 16
    carcass compared with
        goat, 92

    fat characteristics, 3
    heart, 27
    intestine length, 54
    kidney, 63
    liver, 55
    lymph nodes, 35–9
    mouth and tongue, 50
    physiological
        characteristics , 87
    sex characteristics of
        carcass, 91–2
    slaughter, 83
    spleen, 59
    stomach, 52
    teeth, 95
    testicles, 65
    thyroid gland, 76
    tongue, 50
    tonsils, 52
    trachea and lungs, 45
    uterus, 68
    vertebral formula, 12
    see also lamb and mutton
sheep head fly, 158, 161
sheep ked, 158, 160
sheep maggot fly, 158, 160
sheep nostril fly, 158, 160
sheep scab, 163
shell gland, 253
shield, 92
shooting, site of, 82
shotty eruption, 156, 186
shovel beak, 275
Simulium ornatum, 146
Skeletal system, 11–22
    of fowl, 242–5
skeleton
    cow, 13
    fowl, 244
skin, affections of, 186–8
    of fowl, 280
skin tuberculosis, 181
skull, 11
slaughter, 81
    emergency, 85
    of fowl, 256–9
    Jewish, 84
    line, 84
    Muslim, 85
    of rabbit, 231
    ritual, 84, 85, 256
slime, 203

slipped tendons, 272
smell, 102
smoking of bacon, 217
snout, atrophic rhinitis of
    the, 171, 231
snuffles, 233
soft blown cans, 209
somatotrophin, 75
    bovine, 75
sooty mange, 156, 186
sore hocks, 233
spinal cord, 11
spleen, 59
    affections of, 188–9
    of fowl, 250
split aitches, 169
spoilage, canned goods, 208
spondylolisthesis, 275
spondylosis, ankylosing,
    170
Sporotrichum carnis, 165
spotty liver syndrome, 274
springer cans, 209
Spylopsyllus cuniculi, 232
stapes, 74
Staphylococcus aureus, 118
stearin, 3
steatosis, 184
Stephanurus dentatus, 146
stercobilin, 49
sternum, 12
stick marks, 186
'sticking', 83
stomach, 52
    affections of, 189–90
    of fowl, 246
    secretions, 48
strangles, 133
Streptococcus agalactiae,
    183
stress, effects of prolonged,
    106
stunning, 81
    captive bolt, 81
    carbon dioxide, 83
    electric, 82
    mechanical, 81
    of poultry, 256
    of rabbits, 231
sturdy, 150
suffocation, 101
sulphiding, 209

summer mastitis, 183
suprarenal glands, 77
supraspinous ligament, 22
swell, 209
swine erysipelas, 133
swine fever, 134
swine vesicular disease, 135
synasacrum, 243
Syngamus trachea, 268
synovitis, 275
syphilis, rabbit, 223
syrinx, 250

Taenia hydatigena, 149
    ovis, 150
    pisiformis, 151
    saginata, 152
    solium, 152
tail, biting, 187
    necrotic, 187
taint, bone, 103
tapeworms, 146
    cysts in rabbits, 276
    of dogs, 148
    of humans, 151
    of poultry, 276
teeth ageing by, 94–6
    bites, 186–8
    marks, 186
telangiectasis, 176
temperatures, body, 87
tendons, ruptured
    gastrocnemius, 274
Tenuicollis cysts, 149
    tracks, 161
terefah, 85
testes, 65–7
    of fowl, 252
testosterone, 77
tetanus, 135
Thamnidium, 166
thaw rigor, 205
thawing of meat, 205
thermophiles, 202
thick leg disease, 271
thick ropes, 127
thoracic duct, 31
thorax, 14
thrombin, 24
thrombokinase, 24
thrush, 276
thymus, 77

thyroid gland, 76
    cartilage, 43
thyrotrophin, 75
thyroxine, 76
tick pyaemia, 111
ticks, 164
tissue mite nodules, 276
tissues, 2
tongue, 50
    affections of, 170–71
    cooked, 223
    differentiation of, 50–51
    structure, 50
tonsils, 52
toxaemia, 111
    pregnancy, 191
toxins, 113
Toxoplasma gondii, 156
toxoplasmosis, 156
trachea, 43–7
    fowl, 250
transit erythema, 186
transit tetany, 168
traumatic pericarditis, 173
    reticulitis, 189
tread wounds, 276
trematodes, 153
Treponema cuniculi, 223
Trichinella spiralis, 143
trichiniasis, 143
trichinoscope, 144
trichinosis, 143
Trichodectes, 163
Trichophyton, 166
trichophytosis, 166, 187
Trichostrongylus axei, 141
tricuspid valve, 25
tripe, 221
trypsinogen, 49
tuberculosis, 135
    in poultry, 276
    in rabbits, 233
    of bones, 169, 170
    of head and tongue, 170,
        171
    of kidneys, 175
    of livers, 177, 178
    of lungs, 179, 181
    of lymph nodes, 182, 183
    of spleen, 188, 189
    of udders, 183, 184
    skin, 187

Tumours, 192
  in poultry, 277
turkey, 238
turkey rhinotracheitis, 277
twin lamb disease, 191
twisted-leg disease, 277
tympanic membrane, 74
typhoid in fowl, 267
Tyroglyphus farinae, 161
tyrosin crystals, 178

udder, affections of, 183–4
ulcerative enteritis, 277
ulcers
  actinobacillosis, 115
  calf diphtheria, 123
  foot and mouth diseases,
    125
  peptic ulcers, 189
umbilical pyaemia, 177
undulent fever, 123
urachus, 101
uraemia, 167
ureter, 62
urethra, 64
urodeum, 248
urinary organs, 62
urine odour, 167
urogenital system, 62–70
  genital organs, 65–70
  of fowl, 252

uropygeal gland, 241
urticaria, 133
uterus, 67–70
  affections of, 191–2
  of fowl, 253

vagina, 67
  of fowl, 253
vane, 241
veins, 26
venison (see deer and
    venison), 6
venous congestion, 188, 189
ventricle, 25
ventricular furrows, 25
verrucae, 133
verrucose endocarditis, 133
vertebral column, 11
  of fowl, 242
vertebral formulae, 12
vesiculae seminales, 64
viraemia, 111
virus hepatitis of ducks, 277
virus pneumonia, 125
viscera, definition of, 88
visceral gout, fowl, 268
vitamin B_2 deficiency, 265
vitamin B_{12}, 55
vitamin D deficiency, 273
vitelline diverticulum, 247
vitreous humour, 72

warble flies, 158
  larvae, 159
wart, 192
weep, 204
Weil's disease, 128
whiskers, 166
white heifer disease, 191
white muscle, poultry, 245
white spot, 165
white spotted kidney, 175
Wiltshire bacon, 212
winter death syndrome,
    100
wooden tongue, 115
woolsorters' disease (*see*
    anthrax), 116

xanthine, 108
xanthomatosis, 108, 227
xanthophylls, 109
  test for, 105
xanthosis, 108

yeast, 110
yellow fat, 105, 107, 109
  in rabbits, 234
yellow fatted sheep, 109
Yersinia pseudotuberculosis,
    139
  enterolitica, 226
yersiniosis, 139